LOUVAIN PHILOSOPHICAL STUDIES 1

THE BRAIN-MIND PROBLEM

Philosophical and
Neurophysiological Approaches

THE BRAIN-MIND PROBLEM

Philosophical and Neurophysiological Approaches

Contributors
Otto D. CREUTZFELDT
John C. ECCLES
János SZENTÁGOTHAI

Edited by
Balázs GULYÁS

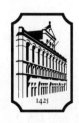

1987
Leuven University Press
Van Gorcum Assen / Maastricht

Acknowledgement is made of the following, who granted permissions to reproduce figures:

The American Physiological Society
Cambridge University Press
R. B. Kelly
P. Roland

Figure 11 on p. 50 is reproduced, with permission, from the Annual Review of Neuroscience, Vol. 2 © 1979 by Annual Reviews Inc.

CIP Koninklijke Bibliotheek Albert I, Brussel.
CIP Koninklijke Bibliotheek, Den Haag

© 1987 Universitaire Pers Leuven / Leuven University Press / Presses Universitaires de Louvain, Krakenstraat 3 - B 3000 Leuven/Louvain, Belgium

ISBN 90 6186 246 9 (Universitaire Pers Leuven)
ISBN 90 232 2318 7 (Van Gorcum)

D/1987/1869/21

Cover: W. Platteborze

CONTENTS

PREFACE

The intention of this interdisciplinary symposium is quite straightforward: to bring into confrontation three famous neuroscientists on a classic philosophical problem, the so-called brain-mind problem. This problem, which historically concerned the relation of body and soul, respectively body and mind, now more specifically concerns the relation of brain and mind. Developments in various areas (the heterogeneous domain called cognitive science, the field of artificial intelligence, and in particular the spectacular progress in brain research made by the neurosciences) open new dimensions to this philosophical problem and provide bases for deeper insights and new questions.

Voltaire, in his criticism of the arrogance of some philosophers, once declared: "Strange! We know not how the earth produces blades of grass; how a woman conceives a child; and yet we pretend to know how ideas are produced!"*

Well, at the present time we have some knowledge of how the earth produces blades of grass, and how a woman conceives a child, but we still are very ignorant of how an idea comes to mind and how symbols can have causal efficacy; we still know very little about what mind is and about its place in nature. But progress toward more satisfactory formulations of the problem and acceptable answers will necessarily have to take into account the spectacular progress of our knowledge in the field of the neurosciences. That is the reason why the confrontation of approaches which this symposium strives for seems particularly promising. And it might perhaps also show that the attitude of some current philosophers who proclaim that the brain-mind problem is essentially solved, or even that it is a pseudo-problem, is a little presumptuous.

Herman Roelants

---

* VOLTAIRE, *Newton versus Leibnitz*, Glasgow, 1764, p. 59.

INTRODUCTION

On the 18th and 19th of April, 1986 a symposium was held in Leuven concerning the brain-mind problem under the auspices of both the Centre for Logic and Philosophy of Science (Head: Professor Herman Roelants) and the Department Brain and Behaviour Research (Head: Professor Marc Callens) of the Catholic University of Leuven. The invited speakers, Otto Creutzfeldt (Göttingen, Germany), Sir John Eccles (Contra, Switzerland), and János Szentágothai (Budapest, Hungary) are all active neuroscientists, who are not only engaged in scientific research, but, as well, are strongly interested in the philosophical problems of their scientific field. The symposium, entitled "The Brain-Mind Problem: Philosophical and Neurophysiological Approaches", provided a platform for the speakers to explain their recent hypotheses, and the opportunity to engage in open discussion with the audience.

This volume presents the papers delivered by the three invited neuroscientists, as well as the transcript of the general discussion.

Leuven
February 3, 1987.

Balázs Gulyás

INEVITABLE DEADLOCKS OF
THE BRAIN-MIND DISCUSSION

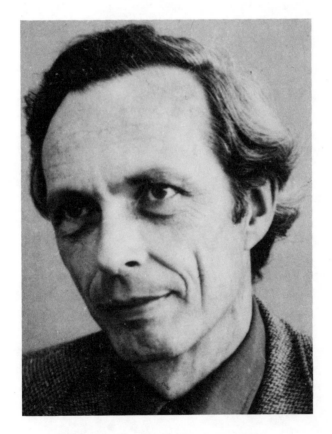

OTTO CREUTZFELDT

Director,
Max-Planck-Institute for Biophysical Chemistry,
Department of Neurobiology,
Am Fassberg, D 3400 Göttingen-Niklausberg, Germany

INTRODUCTION

The relation between mind and body, or between soul and matter, has occupied the human mind since man became aware of himself. But in whatever way men have understood themselves, they have always had difficulty in combining the material (or objective) aspects of their physical existence with the experience of this existence. In religious or in philosophical systems, in one or the other form, we find the idea that mind and body are indeed two different realities, which mutually interact with each other. Different metaphors were used: the soul dwells for a short period in the body and continues after physical death in another body, or as an invisible spirit around us or in another world such as Hades, Heaven or Hell. There is thus an apparent difficulty in accepting that our life is limited and that our conscious experience of life will vanish after death.

In philosophical reasoning we find the idea that mind (or soul, *anima*) and body are related to each other like form and matter (Aristotle)[1], that mind is the (divine) spirit of life in our body (Thomas Aquinas)[30] or that we are dealing with two different forms of matter, a *res extensa* and a *res cogitans* (Descartes)[12]. Thus, although intimately related with each other, both are of a different substance. This again reflects a basic difficulty of the human mind, namely to understand itself only as a product of matter. The human mind had difficulty in accepting such a mechanistic causation, because one of its basic experiences is that it itself causes events by its will and action. How can something "A" be caused by something else "B", if B can be altered by A, with A remaining unaltered? (This is, by the way, the syllogism of the now popular physical mind theories such as expressed by R. Sperry[29], which assume that mind is an emergent property of matter, which — once emerged — gains power over matter.) Would not the foundation of human social behaviour and of human ethics collapse if man accepted the view that he himself, all his actions, all his reasonings and feelings were only a property of matter, however complex? How can values and human ethics result from material interactions?

The difficulty for the human mind in understanding itself simply as a consequence of material events became a scandal only after the scientific revolution of the Renaissance. The human mind was no longer satisfied by a teleological explanation and an understanding of the observed world in the Aristotelian-Scholastic tradition, but wanted to explain it in terms of its causal, mechanistic relationships. It took another 200 years until the "new science" (*nuova sciencia*) of Galilei[18] also tried to explain the human mind. From Aristotle to the modern times, it did not matter where in the body the soul was seated, as long as it was accepted that it was of a different substance and somehow dwelled transiently in the body.

Descartes' location of it into the pineal gland was not so original and only an anatomical detail. Earlier medicine and other cultures had also located the good or bad spirits in the head (and tried to let them out by drilling holes in the skull). But as the new science with its physical laws of gravitation began to replace the spirits, the ethereal forces and the angelic wings that kept the universe together and made the Sun and the planets fly on their courses around the earth, there was eventually no longer a place for the human mind to remain a force or substance not obeying the general laws of nature. If only the same scientific method were applied to the analysis of mind as to the analysis of other phenomena of nature, it should be possible to explain all aspects of human mind and reduce them to physical laws. Then, finally, the ghost could be driven out of the mental machinery[2,11,28].

But in spite of all its efforts and marvellous discoveries, science is yet far from offering a coherent theory of mind, and leaves the answer to the question "What is the nature of mind?" essentially to beliefs. What could be the reason for this? Is it that we are asking the wrong question, or that we are hunting a ghost which does not exist? Or, is the methodological monism of the positivists not applicable to our question? In order to be able to understand this and possibly find an answer to these questions let us now look at some of the details and the impasses the scientific endeavour encounters.

1. THE LOCALIZATION OF MENTAL PROCESSES IN BRAIN STRUCTURES

An essential step in the scientific exploration was that mind is not a single entity or monad, but that it consists of many elements, or mental functions. Philosophers were, of course, for a long time aware of the fact that various mental functions could be distinguished, and that a hierarchy of such mental functions could be established. Such a hierarchy begins at the level of sensations, which are abstracted to ideas (perception), and the various ideas are associated with concepts (cognition) *(Fig. 1)*. Mind is originally a *tabula*

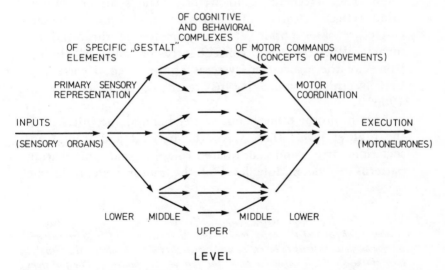

Fig. 1: *A sequential model of cognition, from perception to action. The corresponding "levels" in the brain where the respective processes are supposed to take place are listed at the lower part of the scheme.*

rasa, and develops through the correct combination of sensory elements: *Nihil est in intellectu quod non est in sensu,* as Thomas and later but more elaborately the Empirisists (Hume, Locke) thought.

Neurologists of the 19th and the early 20th centuries discovered that these functions of mind are dependent on the cerebral cortex and that different functions can be disturbed by localised lesions in the various parts or fields of the cerebral cortex *(Fig. 2)*[5,8]. Thus, primary sensations are disturbed by lesions of the "primary" sensory fields, with one available for each sensory function (vision, audition, touch, smell and taste). The higher cognitive functions are disturbed by lesions of the cortical association areas in the parietal lobe, where the sensations of the world around us were supposed to be associated with concepts, leading to what Sigmund Freud had called *"agnosias"*. Such associations did not only refer to ideas of concrete sensory objects or physical events, but also to the combination of abstract symbols, such as calculus and grammar. An association of the sensations of the outside world with those of the inner, subjective world, including emotions, was assumed to be in the prefrontal association cortex. Thus, in 1896, Paul Flechsig could write: "The structure of our mind reflects clearly, in its major subdivisions, the architecture of our brain."[15] And diseases of the mind, or mental illnesses, were consequently pathological disturbances of the association systems of the cerebral cortex, as Carl Wernicke wrote in his textbook of psychiatry in 1906[31].

Action, on the other hand, was elaborated and initiated at the highest level, that is, in the parietal and frontal association cortex, and coordinated to appropriate innervation patterns in the middle level of the motor system, in the

Fig. 2: *The functional cortex map of Kleist (1934). Lesions of various circumscribed parts of the cortex lead to specific functional deficits (from simple sensory or motor deficits to cognitive and personality disturbances). Accordingly, each of these fields is assumed to be the seat of this function. The functions themselves are described in "mental" terms (see text). The numbers refer to the cytoarchitectonic fields according to Brodmann.*

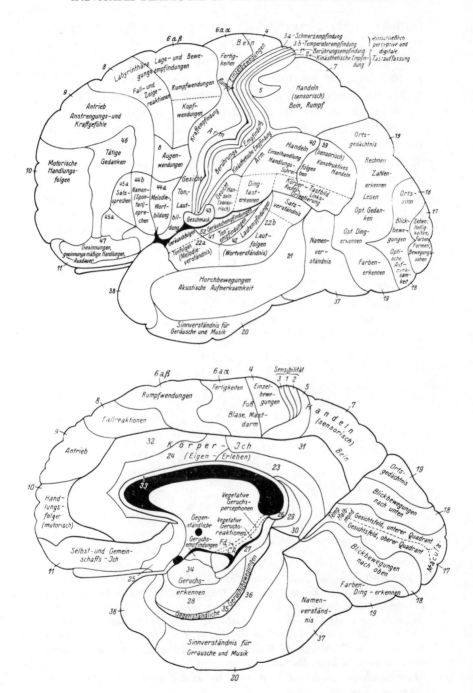

primary motor cortex, which sends its messages for execution to the lowest level, the subcortical and spinal motor nuclei, as Hughling Jackson[22] had concluded at about the same time from neurological observations. In philosophical terms, one may say that the intention to act was elaborated in the highest and the act itself at the middle level.

The linguistic functions of the human mind could be represented in a similar way *(Fig. 3)*. The phonetic elements of language are represented in the primary auditory cortex, and are combined to represent units or words of semantic significance in the sensory speech area of the temporo-parietal association cortex. This in turn may also be considered the highest level for speech production, which is elaborated

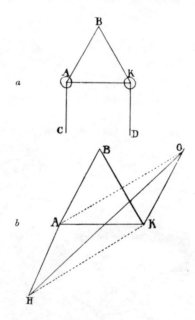

Fig. 3: *Wernicke's classical scheme of of the functional hierarchy of linguistic functions (1894). a) Phonetic signals (D) reach auditory centers (K) in which the speech sounds are supposed to produce activities and memories of sounds, which in turn induce innervation patterns in the speech production centers (A → C). Meanings and ideas are stored in B from where they can be directly formed into words through A. Wernicke did not assume that B was located in one circumscribed area, but that it comprised "the whole cerebral cortex". b) For reading, signals are sent from the visual sphere (H → O) to the language system.*

and transformed into motor programs for speaking in the motor speech area of Broca in the frontal lobe, as Wernicke had concluded from analysis of speech disturbances after circumscribed lesions of the cerebral cortex.

This hierarchical cortical model of perception — sensation — cognition — intention to act — action *(Fig. 1)* was elaborated essentially by the turn of the century, but still prevails in the present day analysis of brain functions. It is easy to recognize that this scheme uses mental descriptions for the functions of mind, which are then projected onto a map of the cerebral cortex.

In the primary sensory and motor fields, i.e., at the middle levels, the sensory surfaces and the muscle systems are indeed layed out as though on maps in topographical order, though with variable scales. These variable scales reflect the significance of the different parts of the respective sensory organs for perception and are expressed already in the sensory periphery by a variable density of sensory nerve cells and/or receptors. It was also assumed that other details of the structure of mind could be revealed by a more exact and more detailed anatomical analysis of the brain, specifically of the cerebral cortex. The morphological and consequently the assumed functional differences among various fields of the cerebral cortex might also reflect their different functions. Could then a complete understanding of the functioning of the various fields and their interactions provide us with the objective categories to describe mind and thus to replace the subjective categories of mental descriptions, the ghost in the machine?

2. ACTIVITIES IN NEURONAL NETWORKS REPRESENT MENTAL PROCESSES

Since the 1950s, neurophysiologists have been able to tap directly with microelectrodes the messages and signals represented in the various sensory and motor fields. They discovered activity patterns of single neurons either elicited by sensory stimuli or during the course of an action. It was found that these signals are related in a straightforward manner to the location, strength and quality of a stimulus *(Fig. 4)*. Even the various elements of a percept were not only represented according to their sensory modality and to their position in the receptor space but also by different neuron classes: colour, texture, countour, orientation of contour or movements of visual objects, the direction of a frequency modulation or the frequency of amplitude modulation of tones, touching the surface of the skin or pinching deeper tissue. These representations of space, modality and quality of a stimulus were not very precisely represented by the individual neurons and the neuronal representations of these various aspects were not independent of each other. Instead, a picture of a neuronal network emerged with relatively few excitatory, but predominantly inhibitory, functional connections between these elements. The functional and spatial parameters of this cortical network were elaborated so that one could, in principle, describe a general algorithm of cortical signal representation (for details see 8). In recent years, the anatomical correlates of this functional network are being uncovered (see Szentágothai, this volume), so that in the near future, we should get a more complete picture of the cortical computational networks which are a necessary condition for representing the elements of perception and action.

The local networks in the sensory fields are not only necessary for perception; their pathological or artificial excitation by focal epileptic discharges or by local electrical

Fig. 4: *Representation of various patterns by the responses of neurons in the visual system (after Creutzfeldt and Nothdurft, 1977). The stimulus patterns are shown in the first row (a). The next rows show what an off- (b) and on-center cell (c) of the lateral geniculate body (LGB) extracts from the various stimuli when scanning the pictures. Note that the LGB-cells transmit to the visual cortex mainly information on contours (last row bird), but that they are also sensitive to the orientation of a line or contour (see middle row, concentric circles). Cortical S-cells (d, e) are strongly orientation-sensitive and each cell represents only incompletely the stimulus pattern. Cortical C-cells (f, g) have a poor spatial resolution, but are sensitive to moving details in a complex stimulus line (SH-cells). In this figure, cell discharges are represented as dots. The pictures are scanned across the receptive fields of the neurons, and discharges are located on that part of the picture which the cell "saw" when discharging.*

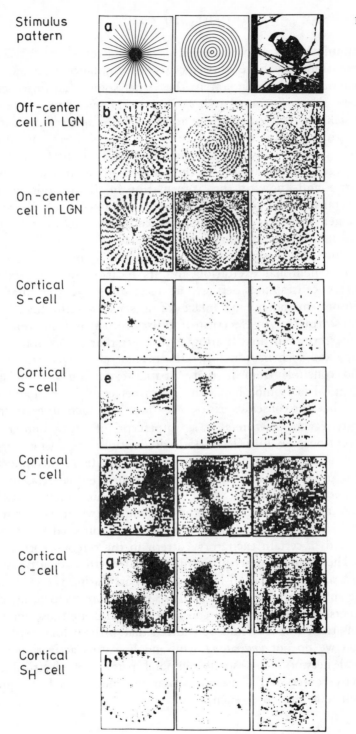

Stimulus pattern

Off-center cell in LGN

On-center cell in LGN

Cortical S-cell

Cortical S-cell

Cortical C-cell

Cortical C-cell

Cortical S$_H$-cell

stimulation is also perceived as a sensation[3,17,25,26]. This sensation may have only a coarse resemblance to a natural stimulus (a flashing star in the visual sphere, an unstructured noise with some pitch quality in the auditory sphere, or a tickling or blunt feeling in the tactile sphere), but it is roughly in the correct place and in the correct modality. This may be considered trivial, knowing all the facts about topographical mapping of the sensory organs in the cerebral cortex and knowing that information in the nervous system is transmitted and represented as excitation of neuronal elements. It has been common knowledge to neurologists and neurosurgeons for over 100 years.

But in the context of our problem it is by no means trivial that a neuronal excitation and its location in the cerebral cortex causes and defines, at least roughly, the quality, sensory modality and place of a sensory stimulus. This transformation of electrical impulses into sensations remains a mystery. But does it allow us to state that the excitation of such and such neurons "*is*" the percept of a given stimulus, and conclude from it that "spatial excitation patterns are identical or isomorphic with certain percepts"? Or should we say that our conscious experience "*looks*" at such an excitatory pattern and interprets it as a percept, if other borderline conditions are fullfilled? Both descriptions are metaphorical and as such scientifically correct. The dualistic metaphor is also used by neurophysiologists, whom we may classify as physicalists, such as R. Jung[23], P. Changeaux[4] or F. Crick[10], who talk about the searchlight of attention (whatever this may be in neurophysiological terms) which is directed or turned towards a certain excitatory pattern in the cerebral cortex.

The monistic description may be satisfactory for a physical *explanation,* because all biophysical events during the sensation are sufficiently described. If there is no more happening, the events described may be considered a sufficient cause for the sensation. But it should be realized that with such an explanation we do not *understand* why and how this activation of a local network, this spatio-temporal pattern of electrical activity, enters our conscious sensation (and is, in fact, quite well remembered as such).

Our problem becomes more complicated if we look at further details. We have learned, during the last 10 or 15 years, that each sensory organ is not only represented once or twice in the cerebral cortex, but up to 10 times or more *(Fig. 5)* (for details see 8). This means that a given stimulus not only excites one set of neurons in the respective sensory field of the cerebral cortex, but many sets. Each of these sets, however, is activated in a different manner and by a different combination of details of a complex stimulus. Thus, in some sets of neurons in these additional sensory areas, different features of a stimulus may be more strongly represented than in other sets, for example, movement of a visual object, or its texture or colour. On the other hand, the exact location of a stimulus in visual space or in the auditory system, along the frequency scale, is

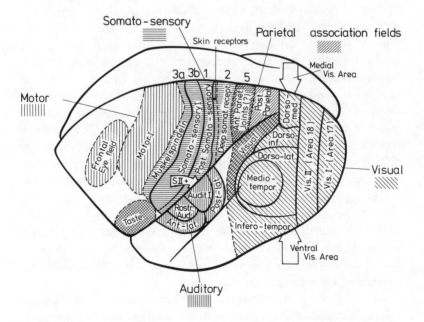

Fig. 5: *Multiple representation of sensory surfaces in the cortex (after All-mann, Merzenich and Kaas, 1977-1980). The various visual fields are marked with diagonal, the auditory fields with vertical and the somato-sensory fields with horizontal hatching. In this map, 10 visual, 4 auditory and 5 somato-sensory fields are distinguished.*

much less precise than in the respective primary area. Thus, coactivation of a set of neurons in one or several of the additional spatially less precise sensory areas adds a specific label to the sensory activation in the respective primary area[9].

Lesion of such areas may produce, in man, various forms of cognitive defects (agnosias). Activation of these labelling sets alone, on the other hand, may not produce a sensation at all, or — if it does — only crude sensations that are difficult for the subject to interpret and to describe. In areas that are necessary for a more complex sensory analysis such as the sensory speech area (Wernicke's area), local excitation such as elicited by focal electrical stimulation will interfere with the understanding of language or with finding the right word for an object (anomia), but such circumscribed excitation will not elicit even the crudest sensation of linguistic elements or anything else.

The same applies to focal excitations in the parietal association cortex, although neurons in this area are excitable by sensory stimuli. This region is, in various ways, involved in relating sensory inputs to appropriate motor commands[20], or more generally to an appropriate intention to act. Lesion of such areas makes a person unable to understand the meaning of an object and to use it appropriately. It produces, in neurological terms, various forms of agnosias and apraxias. The person sees or hears or feels correctly, but this sensation cannot be related to ideas and action schemes. One may therefore say that the activation of a set of neurons in the parietal association cortex represents a functional relationship between the world around the individual[16] and with his repertoire of interaction with this world, i.e., how he relates himself actively to this world. But activation of such sets of neurons by electrical or pathological excitation is again not perceived. "Ideas without sensations are empty", as Kant said.

At the next level, the level of action itself, i.e., the motor cortex, excitations of circumscribed sets of neurons produce contractions of single or neighbouring muscles. If the spatio-temporal coordination of different sets is appropriate, coordinated movements can result, as these sets are connected directly or indirectly (via motor nuclei in the midbrain) to the motor neurons of the lower brain stem and the spinal cord, i.e., the final common path. But the subject experiences only the effect of these activities, i.e., the contractions of the muscles, but no intention to move. The neurons in the motor cortex also get sensory input from skin receptors for feedback control of the force to be engaged to overcome or compensate for resistances in the path of the movement. But these sensory messages are not experienced when the motor cortex is excited directly either by an epileptic discharge or an electrical stimulation. Electrical stimulation or epileptic discharges in the premotor cortex or the supplementary motor area produce more coordinated, synergistic contractions of many, predominantly proximal muscles, but again no intention to move or any other sensation.

If the motor speech area in front of the motor cortex (Broca's area) is stimulated by electrical stimulation or pathological discharges, the subject simply interrupts a speech sequence for the time of the excitation, but does not know why, and neither speech sounds nor subjective experiences are elicited.

I mentioned these various examples to demonstrate that excitation of circumscribed sets of neurons in the cerebral cortex does not necessarily reach conscious experience. In fact, only the activity of a very small minority of neurons in the sensory areas can be said to "cause" sensations because many of the cortical neurons only function to inhibit others. A further qualification is necessary, if it is realized that neurons are active continually: only certain changes of their activity relative to the activity of others surrounding them causes a sensation.

The activation of the large majority of cortical neurons is not experienced as such, but represents certain functional relations of the sensations to intentional models, intentions to act or actual movements[9]. Recording their activity is like recording the potentials from a functional module in a computer which does a certain transformation of a number or a set of numbers, say transforming a number into its logarithm, or angular degrees into their sine or cosine. Potentials in such a module only tell the investigator that such a transformation is being performed, without telling him the input or the output numbers. These can only be seen on the video-screen of the computer, and are meaningful only if the transform function is known to the observer.

One may apply this comparison and use it for our argument. One could then say that only the activity patterns of some neurons in some areas of the cerebral cortex are the screens for conscious perception. This conscious perception "knows" the functional significance or transformation of these patterns, because other sets or patterns of activity are coactivated and thus enable conscious perception to incorporate within itself a model of the world and of its interaction with this world. It is indeed difficult to avoid dualistic metaphors if one tries to describe and to understand what is going on in our brain during perception.

Whereas most of the activity patterns of the brain are not perceived as such, the subject can clearly induce them. One can train even a monkey to increase or decrease the discharge rate of a neuron in its motor cortex, if it is allowed to listen to the discharge rate and if it is rewarded for keeping the activity on a certain level[14]. In humans, it is possible to make the gross activity of circumscribed cortical regions "visible" by measuring the cerebral blood flow (rCBF)[21] or the glucose metabolism (with PET)[19]. If, for example, a person is asked to imagine his living room and to name all the objects which he sees there, or if he is asked to perform an imaginary walk from one place to another, activation is found in the various brain regions which are involved in the execution of such a task[27]. Thus, a person can voluntarily, i.e., by his own free will, make certain areas of his brain work (although this activity is not experienced when elicited by itself). Only if the subject is a good neurologist and knows which area is involved in which task can he think of the right task and thus hope that the area he wishes to activate will "work". Here again, would it be unscientific and incorrect to use the metaphor and to say that the subject "makes" certain areas of his brain work? This metaphor is incorrect only insofar as the subject does not activate a certain area of the brain like he moves a finger, because there is no indication to him that the area is activated, and all he knows is that he performs a certain mental task. But not all neurons in all parts of the cortex can be activated by the subject from inside. If, for example, recordings are taken from a neuron which is activated or inhibited when the subject speaks aloud, because its activity is modulated by the speech of the subject, this neuron is not activated by internal maneuvers such as silent speech or silent reading *(Fig. 6)*.

NAMES PICTURES.   SILENT NAMING

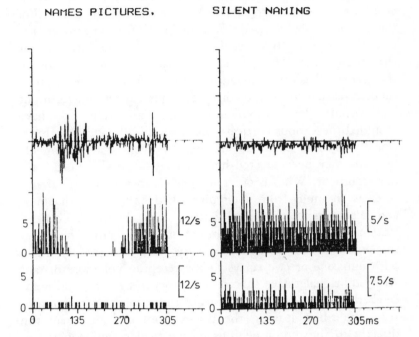

Fig. 6: *Averaged activity of a cortical neuron in the right temporal lobe (superior temporal gyrus) of a human person while he names an object (left) and when he names the object silently (Creutzfeldt and Ojemann, to be published). First line of recording: microphone record of the subject's speech. At time zero a drawing of a simple object is shown to the patient. Second and third lines: averaged activity of two simultaneously recorded neurons. The neuron in the top record is inhibited during and following the word pronunciation (left), but the activity does not change when the subject names the object only in his mind (right, silent naming). (x-axis: time in milliseconds, y-axis: response in number of spikes)*

We may conclude, simplifying somewhat, that only neurons in those regions of the brain which are involved in actions or in intentions to act can be voluntarily activated by performing the appropriate maneuvers, while neurons in predominantly sensory regions, the activation of which causes sensations, cannot be activated internally, but only by the appropriate input from the respective sensory organ.

3. THE BRAIN AS A CONTROL SYSTEM

If we consider the brain just as a control system, which enables the organism to survive in its environment, a model of the brain can be devised, in principle. With regard to the cerebral cortex, such a model would have to take into account that the principal functional and anatomical organization of the cortex is basically universal and that the functional significance of each part of the cortex depends entirely on its input and output[7]. These input and output connections may have moulded the various cortical areas anatomically and even functionally to some extent during their ontogenetic development, but this may be neglected here as it is of no significance for our argument. What is of significance is that each cortical area receives an input from a circumscribed part of the thalamus and sends its cortico-fugal output into the motor control systems of the lower brainstem or the spinal cord. The thalamic input to one area may be very close to a sensory organ with only one or two relays to the receptors, or more distant with additional relays in cerebral structures of the midbrain, cerebellum or even some regions of the cortex. On the output side, the fibres leaving the cortex from one area may run directly to the motor neurons of the final common path, or

Fig. 7: *Schematic representation of a cortical model of parallel input-output loops. A: Each loop has an input line from the thalamus and is more or less directly activated from a circumscribed region of a sensory surface. After processing in the local intracortical network, the output feeds more or less directly into subcortical or spinal motor control systems. Thus, each local sensory input induces a local response, i.e., a movement or an intention to move. The cortex consists of a myriad of such parallel input-output loops (A...C...Z). B: Through intracortical spread of afferent fibres (A...C), short range ($\alpha...\beta$) and long range ($\alpha...\varkappa...\omega$) intercortical connections, these loops are interconnected with each other in variable ways. C: Also at lower, subcortical levels connections exist between the loops (via the basal ganglia, in the brainstem motor nuclei, the medullary and spinal motoneuron pools etc.). Here, the various impulses for movements are integrated into an appropriate motor response. D: Each motor response, whether executed or only intended, leads to a different position (or intended position) of the subject relative to his environment (a--a', b--b' etc.). As a consequence, the sensory input elicited by the environment changes, and there is no static representation of the environment in the brain (open loop).*

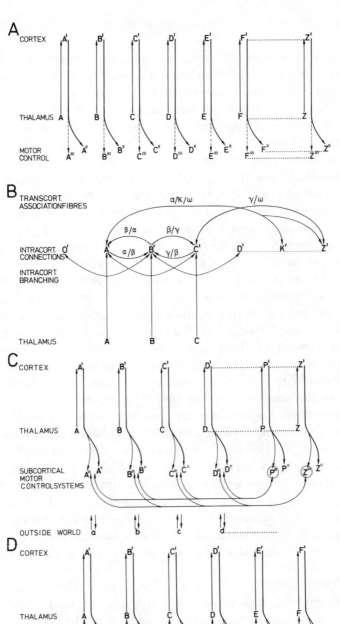

may terminate in subcortical motor control stations such as the motor nuclei of the brainstem, the tectum or cerebellum.

With this qualification, the cortex may be considered as a system of a myriad of parallel loops, each of them being excited more or less directly by some outside (sensory) signal and each transforming this outside excitation more or less directly into an impulse for action *(Fig. 7)*[8]. This may be illustrated by a few examples: local electrical or sensory excitation of a set of cells in the cortical representation of the peripheral visual field in the primary visual area will induce an eye movement with the intention to fixate this object on the fovea; neurons in extrastriate (i.e., secondary) visual fields are not only activated by visual stimuli but also when the subject intends to respond to the stimulus by looking at it; in the parietal association cortex, neurons are "sensory" as they can be excited by sensory stimuli (and have "receptive fields"), but are also "motor" in that they are active before a movement starts; in the primary motor cortex the activation of neurons is causally related to the contraction of muscles, but their activity is — as we mentioned — also under the control of somatosensory receptors (mainly pressure receptors in the skin), which are the necessary peripheral sensors of an effective, force-controlling feedback loop (for details and further references see 8, 9). (We will, in this context, disregard the horizontal interactions between these various vertical loops through short- and long-ranging association fibers. Their functional significance is not yet completely understood. It should be pointed out, however, that their course does not always follow the hierarchical mental scheme from sensation to action, which we had mentioned earlier. But it would lead us too far, to elaborate on this).

These cortical input-output loops thus relate, each in a different way, the subject with the outside world, and thus change or intend to change the relation of the subject to the world. In this way, there is no single stable state between the subject (or his brain) and his inner or outer environment as each new position entails a different input which causes another new position, and so on.

In this manner, the brain has become a perfect control system, the purpose of which is to keep the subject and the species alive. In such a control system we may incorporate drives, emotions, memory, fatigue and even some type of spontaneity, but we do not need consciousness, i.e., reflective self-awareness of the various relations of the subject to his world, as long as the machine works perfectly. As observers, we can sufficiently *explain* this system if we have a complete knowledge of its anatomical and functional connections, of its sensors and tools, and of its modifiability by various states of drive. But in order to *understand* it, we need to know its purpose, that means a teleological explanation (the distinction of *explanation* and *understanding* is used here as defined by Wright[33]).

The same applies to any control system: it is easy to explain the working of a thermostat (in physical terms) by analysing its elements, but to understand it one needs a teleological explanation, a knowledge of its purpose. The machine itself does not need to know its purpose in order to function as designed. Nor does an ant need to know the hierarchy and the purpose of the complicated organization of an ant society in order to fulfill its purpose within it. It is a principal mistake often made when discussing artificial or animal intelligence to assume that the subject must be aware of his existence and of the purpose of his behaviour. A robot can do its job without knowing that and why it is doing it.

4. CONDITIONS OF MIND

In explaining and understanding a control system, be it technical or biological, we would never expect to discover the "mind" of that system. We may at best admire the mastermind behind it, the wisdom of the designer or the wisdom of nature if we recognize that the design is consistent with the purpose of that machine. In the case of biological organisms this purpose is determined by our view of nature, and it is typically reduced to the finite survival of the individual and the unlimited survival of the species in a given environment. Our scientific education makes us accept the fact that there is life as defined scientifically, and we may even explain its origin and continuation, but we consider the question "why and for what purpose is life?" as unscientific, and therefore illegitimate and inappropriate. In such reasoning one might, however, accept the notion of mind and use this word as a mental description of operational intelligence.

Mind implies, however, that the subject is aware of himself and of his existence in this world. This awareness will lead sooner or later to the "inappropriate" questions: what are the conditions of my existence, of the world, of my interactions with this world and with other individuals? It will necessarily lead to the further question of the purpose and goal of our existence, the existential questions. To say that these questions are unscientific does not mean that they are wrong or non-existent[32]. It only means that science cannot give explanations to answer them.

This questioning certainly starts in our brain, and there must be a mechanism which actually makes it possible. This mechanism must be closely linked to the ability of our brain to be aware and to symbolize what is represented to it, and the actions which it intends or does. Through these symbols man relates himself to himself, to others and to the world. In these symbols he unifies the distributed activities of his brain, and presents them back to himself, in what we may call the *reflective loop*[6]. But these symbols are not the physical reality of the world, nor are they identical with the activities of the brain. They become a reality in themselves; we relate to them and they influence our lives and affect our brains as much as or even more than the physical world around us. Through these symbols, the brain transcends its own functions and becomes able to reason about itself, about human existence, about the world and the relation of itself to this world — and this reasoning will lead to questions which it cannot answer. It is not satisfied by causal explanations, but wants to understand.

CONCLUSIONS

Where has our attempt to look at some relations between brain and mind led us? We have started with the hypothesis that there may be an isomorphic relationship between brain activities and mental processes (cf. 13). We referred to the classical neurological schemes which in one way or another inserted mental schemes of mind from perception, cognition, and action onto brain maps. We could verify some aspects of this hypothesis by analysing effects of electrical brain stimulation, focal epileptic excitations or lesions. But we also found that already at such a basic level, the experience and description of the sensations thus elicited cannot avoid using a dualistic terminology. We concluded from this that duality may be an essential feature of conscious experience.

We furthermore realized that activities in certain parts of the cerebral cortex will only represent operational processes involved in functional connections (or associations) between certain neuronal representation but will not enter consciousness as such. We also realized that activities of some regions do not at all elicit conscious experience as such but only the somatic effects of their activities, such as muscle contractions. These observations do not necessarily violate the hypothesis of isomorphism, but entail complex assumptions. They are not consistent with the simple declaration that conscious experience is a feature of neuronal activities in the cerebral cortex. This would also have to be qualified. But, however qualified, the fact that the electrical discharge patterns of certain neurons enter consciousness, and that their location within the brain adds space and quality to that activity, is a mystery which we cannot explain.

We then considered the brain simply as a control system. We looked at the cortex as a structure consisting of a myriad of parallel input-output loops from sensory to action systems, some of them with direct access to sensory inputs but more indirect access to outputs, others with more direct access to motor outputs, and some in between. In this way the cortex actively relates the subject in various ways to the environment by responses which may be directly translated into movement through lower motor integrating systems, or by causing intentions to move (or, as the neurophysiologist would say, by facilitating motor impulses).

In this sense, sensation and action are ubiquitous properties of the cortex with variable emphasis on one or the other in the various fields. Although such a model can, in principle, explain behaviour, we realized that it does not explain nor does it need conscious experience. But we can conclude from such a model, which is based on anatomical and physiological data, that the design of brain machinery is not the same as the design deduced from the mental description of our reasoning. The machinery of the brain uses parallel input-output lines, while the mental schemes assume a system of serial processing. From this we must conclude that mental processes as we understand them are not isomorphic with the processes in the brain. Blackbox models are not sufficient explanations.

At the next step we realized that a necessary condition for mind is conscious experience. This is a single experience[24], and therefore must integrate the various distributed activities across the cerebral cortex to a single sensation. We can describe this only by a dualistic metaphor such as: all the various activities in the myriads of sensori-motor loops are integrated and appear on a single video-screen, at which the subject looks. This dualistic metaphor must not, of course, be taken as a proof of a Cartesian dualism. But it indicates that any sensible description of the relation between mind and brain gets trapped in such a dualistic terminology, which therefore must be considered a specific feature of reasoning.

We then argued that the other condition for mind is the ability of the brain to transform its own states, the states of the world around it as well as the relation between the subject and his world, into symbols of such states. It can re-represent these symbols to itself in a reflective loop and also communicate them to others. These symbols are not the real world, but they allow a consistent description of it and of our relation to it. Our conscious reasoning is therefore not identical with brain activities, but with the symbolic significance or the meaning of these activities in the context of a system of symbols. But as the symbols carry significant information, they are a reality. They are the language of our reason and therefore the language of our mind.

We then realized that reason is not satisfied by causal explanations; it wants to understand and for that it needs teleological explanations. These cannot be given by science, which only gives causal explanations. Here the Aristotelian and the Galilean argumentation, teleology vs. positivism, clash. We are at an impasse: "Our reason has this peculiar fate that, with reference to one class of its knowledge, it is always troubled with questions which cannot be ignored, because they spring from the very nature of reason, and which cannot be answered, because they transcend the powers of human reason," as Kant put it in the first sentence of the Preface to his *Critique of Pure Reason*[24].

This was the path of our argumentation. Our conclusions should not be misunderstood, however, as indicating that the scientific reasoning or the methodological monism of positivism, the universality of which we challenged at the beginning, is inappropriate for analyzing the machinery which enables us to ask these questions. Scientific reasoning is the only way to keep our world of mind, our world of symbols, our models of the world including those of our brains and its functions, as close to reality as possible. This is the promise of science, and the only way for mankind after it has picked the fruits of scientific cognition. But scientific reasoning must see its limits and should not pretend to be able to answer questions which "transcend its abilites". Otherwise it will reintroduce the ghosts which it claims to drive out.

REFERENCES:

1. ARISTOTLE, *De Anima.*
2. BIERL, P. (1981). *Analytische Philosophie des Geistes.* Konigstein, Ts.: Hain.
3. CALVIN, W.H. and OJEMANN, G.A. (1980). *Inside the Brain.* New York: New American Library.
4. CHANGEUX, P. (1983). *L'homme neuronal.* Paris: Fayard.
5. CLARKE, E. and DEWHORST, K. (1973). *Die Funktionen des Gehirns. Lokalisationstheorien von der Antike bis zur Gegenwart.* München: Heinz Moos Verlag.
6. CREUTZFELDT, O. (1979). Neurophysiological Mechanisms and Consciousness. In: *Brain and Mind,* CIBA Foundation Series 69. Amsterdam: Elsevier-North Holland, pp. 217-233.
7. CREUTZFELDT, O. (1977). Generality of the Functional Structure of the Neocortex. *Naturwissenschaften* 64: 507-517.
8. CREUTZFELDT, O. (1983). *Cortex Cerebri. Leistung, strukturelle und funktionelle Organisation der Hirnrinde.* Berlin-Heidelberg-New York: Springer.
9. CREUTZFELDT, O. (1986). Comparative Aspects of Representation in the Visual System. In: *Pattern Recognition Mechanisms. Study Week of the Pontifical Academy of Sciences,* C. CHAGAS and R. GATTAS (eds.). Exp. Brain Res., Suppl. 11, pp. 53-82.
10. CRICK, F. (1984). Function of the Thalamic Reticular Complex: The Search Light Hypothesis. *Proc. Natl. Acad. Sci.* 81: 4586-4590.
11. DENNETT, D.C. (1969). *Brain Storms. Philosophical Essays on Mind and Psychology.* Hassockx, Suss.: Harvester Press.
12. DESCARTES, R. (1664). *De homine.*
13. FEIGL, H. (1959). *The "Mental" and the "Physical".* Minneapolis, Miss.: University of Minnesota Press.
14. FETZ, E., Personal communication.
15. FLECHSIG, P. (1896). *Die Localisation der geistigen Vorgang, insbesondere der Sinnesempfindungen des Menschen.* Leipzig.
16. FLEICHSIG, P. (1896). *Gehirn und Seele.* 2. Aufl. Leipzig.
17. FOERSTER, O. (1936). Motorische Felder und Bahnen. In: *Handbuch der Neurologie,* vol. VI, O. BUMKE and O. FOERSTER (eds.). Berlin-Heidelberg-New York: Springer, pp. 1-357.
18. GALILEI, G. (1638). *Discorsi e dimostrazioni matematiche intorno a' due nuove scienze.*
19. HEISS, W.-D. (1985). Hirnfunktionen sichtbar gemacht. *Die Positron-Emissions-Tomographie als eine Methode diagnostischer Stoffwechseluntersuchungen.* Max-Planck-Gesellschaft, pp. 36-56.
20. HYVARINEN, J. (1982). *The Parietal Cortex of Monkey and Man.* Berlin-Heidelberg-New York: Springer.
21. INGVAR, D. and LASSEN, N.A. (eds.), *Brain Work: The Coupling of Function, Metabolism and Blood Flow in the Brain.* Copenhagen: Munksgaard.

22. JACKSON, J.H. (1931). *Selected Writings of John Hughlings Jackson.* 2 vols. London: Hodder and Stoughton. Reprinted in New York: Basic Books Inc., 1958.

23. JUNG, R. (1978). Perception, Consciousness and Visual Attention. In: *Central Correlates of Conscious Experience,* P. BUSER and A. ROUGEUL-BUSER (eds.). Amsterdam: Elsevier-North Holland, pp. 15-36.

24. KANT, I. (1781). *Critik der reinen Vernunft.* English translation by F.M. Müller, New York: Anchor Books, 1966.

25. PENFIELD, W. (1958). *The Excitable Cortex in Conscious Man.* Liverpool: Liverpool University Press.

26. PENFIELD, W. and RASMUSSEN, T. (1958). *The Cerebral Cortex of Man.* New York: MacMillan.

27. ROLAND, P. and FRIBERG, L. (1985). Localization of Cortical Areas Activated by Thinking. *J. Neurophysiol.* 53: 1219-1243.

28. RYLE, G. (1949). *The Concept of Mind.* London: Hutchinson.

29. SPERRY, R. (1980). Mind-Brain Interaction: Mentalism, Yes; Dualism, No. *Neurosciences* 5: 195-206.

30. THOMAS AQUINAS. *Summa Theologiae* I: qq. 75-76.

31. WERNICKE, C. (1906). *Grundriss der Psychiatrie,* H. LIPEMANN (ed.), Leipzig: Thieme.

32. WITTGENSTEIN, L. (1961). *Tractus logico-philosophicus.* (6.371) New York: Routledge and Kegan Paul.

33. WRIGHT von, G.H. (1984). *Erklaren und Verstehen.* Königstein, Ts.: Athenaum Verlag.

THE EFFECT OF SILENT THINKING ON THE CEREBRAL CORTEX

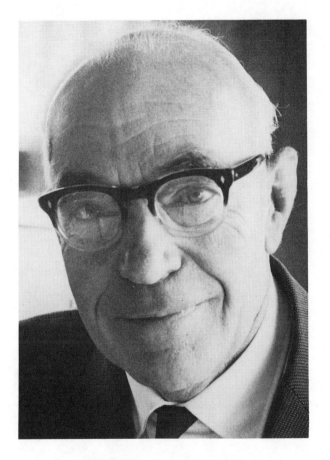

JOHN C. ECCLES

Emeritus Professor,
Recipient of the Nobel Prize in
Physiology and Medicine (1963),
CH 6611 Contra (TI), Switzerland

1. THINKING

With the exception of the hard-core radical materialists
there is general agreement on the existence of mental events
such as thinking. Thinking is, of course, subjectively experienced and is not objectively identifiable in the way that
we perceive the world around us through our senses. Popper
has sharpened this distinction by his classification of the
whole world of matter-energy as World 1 and the world of
subjective experience as World 2. A test of such a division is
provided by the analysis of such experiences as illusions and
hallucinations, which, though interpreted by the ex-
periencer as being in World 1, have to be recognized as
being in World 2. For example, the apparently objective
world of a dream experience has in fact no World 1 status,
but is entirely in World 2. Of course, simultaneously with
the dream, objective World 1 happenings can be recognized
in the brain and even in the body of the dreamer, but they
give no evidence of the content of the dream as recounted on
awakening.

There are wide ranges of mental events as illustrated in
the World 2 list in *Fig. 1,* but all can be subsumed under
the general term "mind", which is again in general philosophical use after its eclipse by Ryle's great, cathartic book
The Concept of Mind[28]. The recovery is signalled by such
books as *The Existence of Mind* by Beloff[4] and *Content and
Consciousness* by Dennett[7], where it is stated that "the most
central feature of mind, the 'phenomenon' that seems more
than any other to be quintessentially 'mental' and non-phy-
sical is consciousness" (p. 99). In their book *The Self and Its
Brain*[23] Popper and Eccles give equal status to World 1 and
World 2, a dualism as sharp as that of Descartes, and are
specially concerned with the problem of interactionism.

Finally, in his book *The Nature of Mind,* Armstrong[3],
though still regarding himself as a physicalist, presents a

most insightful account of consciousness and introspection stating that "without introspective consciousness there would be little or no memory of the past history of the self — we would not be aware that we existed" (p. 68).

In *Fig. 1* "thinking" is listed as one of the subjective experiences in World 2. It is a word covering an immense range of mental happenings. In order to limit philosophical discussion Beloff[4] defines thinking "as the activity of problem solving" (p. 98), but he immediately enlarges the scope by stating that a problem exists whenever some *end* is sought, but the *means* to that end has still to be discovered. That definition is too narrow for our present purpose where the thinking is mental concentration that usually is on some particular learnt program or algorithm, but which also may be mental concentration on some anticipated sensory input. Thus we can limit our concept of thinking to *mental concentration on some particular task.* Philosophical discussion on the concept of thinking and the brain-mind problem will follow an account of the extraordinary findings on human brains engaged in thinking that is related to a variety of learnt procedures. In this way it comes about that there is an internal generation of thinking in the absence of any signalling to the brain by sense organs.

2. CEREBRAL EVENTS DURING THINKING

Fig. 2 shows the brain (cerebral cortex) in the head with the rather arbitrary division into the four lobes, frontal, parietal, temporal and occipital, with the primary visual, auditory, somatosensory and motor areas indicated. This will serve as a basic cortical map for orientation of the areas activated in various types of silent thinking. *Fig. 3* gives a diagrammatic representation of the extremely complicated

Fig. 1: *Tabular representation of the contents of the three worlds that comprise everything in existence and in experience.*

WORLD 1

PHYSICAL OBJECTS AND STATES

1. INORGANIC

Matter and energy of cosmos

2. BIOLOGY

Structure and actions
of all living beings
- human brains

3. ARTEFACTS

Material substrates
of human creativity
of tools
of machines
of books
of works of art
of music

WORLD 2

STATES OF CONSCIOUSNESS

Subjective knowledge

Experience of
perception
thinking
emotions
dispositional intentions
memories
dreams
creative imagination

WORLD 3

KNOWLEDGE IN OBJECTIVE SENSE

Cultural heritage coded
on material substrates
philosophical
theological
scientific
historical
literary
artistic
technological

Theoretical systems
scientific problems
critical arguments

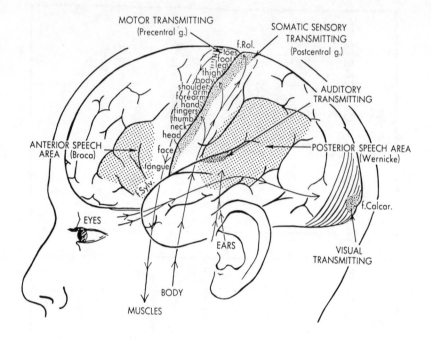

Fig. 2: *The motor and sensory transmitting areas of the cerebral cortex. The approximate map of the motor transmitting areas is shown in the precentral gyrus, while the somatic sensory areas are in a similar map in the postcentral gyrus. Actually the toes, foot and leg should be represented over the top of the medial surface. Other primary sensory areas shown are the visual and auditory, but they are largely in areas screened from this lateral view. The frontal, parietal, occipital and temporal lobes are indicated. Also shown are the speech areas of Broca and Wernicke.*

procedures used for measuring the regional cerebral blood flow (rCBF) during thinking[24,25,26]. With present techniques the spatial resolving power of the radioactive Xenon (^{133}Xe) technique is no better than 1.0 cm^2. The rCBF can be assumed to be a reliable indicator of the neuronal activity in that area. An assemblage of 254 collimator tubes over one cerebral hemisphere recorded the emission from the ^{133}Xe in the cerebral circulation for 45 seconds after the 1 second long injection of the solution into the internal carotid artery *(Fig. 3)*. *Fig. 3* indicates in a greatly simplified form the steps whereby there is an integration and synthesis of the data from the 254 assemblage into a rCBF map of the

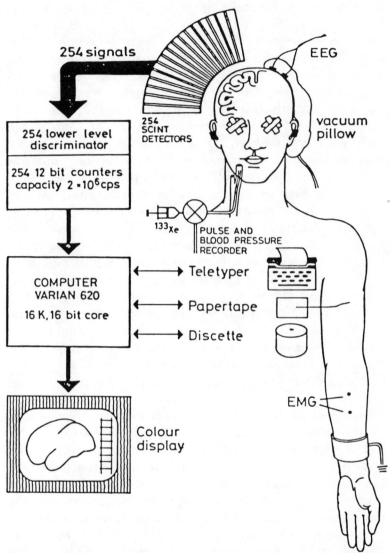

254 signals

EEG

254 lower level discriminator

254 12 bit counters capacity 2 • 10⁶cps

254 SCINT DETECTORS

vacuum pillow

133Xe

PULSE AND BLOOD PRESSURE RECORDER

COMPUTER VARIAN 620

16 K, 16 bit core

Teletyper

Papertape

Discette

EMG

Colour display

Fig. 3: *Block diagram of the equipment and the principles of the method. The head is fixed to the collimator by a vacuum pillow. The 254 collimator tubes are arranged radially in a 50 mm-thick spherical lead segment. The spatial resolving power of the camera when used for rCBF measurements is one channel. The center-to-center distance of 2 adjacent collimator tubes is 10 mm. Signals from the 254 cortical regions are processed on-line, the isotope clearance curves, the rCBF values, and background radioactivity can be recorded in the three different formats for further processing or displayed on the TV-screen (Roland et al., 1980)*[26].

subjacent cerebral cortex. The technique necessarily involves the very coarse temporal grain of 45 to 60 seconds, which is the time for clearance of the ^{133}Xe from the cerebral blood flow. When determining the rCBF for some specific cerebral action, it is essential to allow for the background activity as indicated by the rCBF of the cerebral cortex when the subject is literally thinking of nothing. In the rCBF maps here illustrated this allowance has always been made, and moreover there has been a synthesis of several experimental runs on the same or other subjects with calculation of the statistical significances of the percentage increases. It is remarkable that in all the diverse experimental tests no significant rCBF reduction of any area was ever observed.

Fig. 4 illustrates a remarkable finding of Roland[24] that when the human subject was attending with concentration to a finger on which just detectable touch stimuli were to be applied, there was an increase in the rCBF over the finger touch area of the postcentral gyrus of the cerebral cortex (Fig. 2) as well as in the mid-prefrontal area. These increases must have resulted from the mental attention because actually no touch was applied during the recording. Thus, Fig. 4 is a clear demonstration that the mental act of concentrated attention (thinking) can activate appropriate regions of the cerebral cortex. A similar finding occurs with attention to the lips in expectation of a touch, but of course the activated somatosensory area is now for the lips.

The effect of concentrated attention in causing an increased cerebral electrical response to finger touch has also been demonstrated by Desmedt and Robinson[8]. In a very ingenious investigation they discovered that, with touch to the attended finger, there was a large increase in the late N 140 and P 500 waves of the evoked potentials relative to controls with touch to unattended fingers. This may be correlated with the increased rCBF that attention produced in the finger area of Fig. 4. In both of these investigations the concentrated attention or thinking was effecting selective neuronal responses.

More recently Roland and Fiberg[25] have carried out a similar investigation on more complex thinking procedures. The subject had to learn these procedures by repeated re-

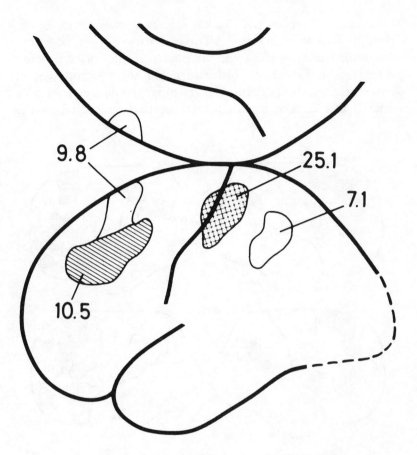

Fig. 4: *Mean increase of rCBF in percent during pure selective somatosensory attention; that is, somatosensory latent sensing without peripheral stimulation. The size and location of each focus shown is the geometrical average of the individual focus. Each individual focus has been transferred to a brain map of standard dimensions with a proportional stereotaxic system. The cross-hatched areas have an increase of rCBF significant at the 0.00005 level (Student's test, one-sided significance level). For the other areas shown the rCBF increase is significant at the 0.05 level. Eight subjects. (Roland, 1981)*[24]

hearsal. Thus in all cases there is a background of instructional indoctrination, but it always ceased well before the experimental run with the injected [133]Xe. The subject is lying with eyes and ears closed (cf. *Fig. 3)* and is at complete rest with no muscular movements except for quiet

breathing. This is the background on which the silent
thinking is superimposed. Three distinct types of silent
thinking were investigated, the pooled results of each being
displayed in *Fig. 5.* In order to avoid the development of
automatic responses the initial training procedures were on a
related but different paradigm from that presented to the

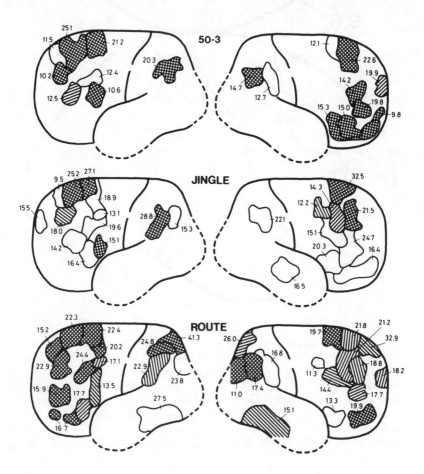

Fig. 5: *Mean increases of rCBF in percent and their average distribution in
cerebral cortex under three different conditions of silent thinking as described in
the text. Left hemisphere six subjects, right hemisphere five subjects. Cross-hatched areas have rCBF increases significant at the 0.005 level. With hatched
areas P < 0.01 and with outlined areas P < 0.05 (Roland and Friberg,
1985)*[25].

subject some time (> 27 sec) before the actual experimental run.

In *Fig.* 5 the 50-3 frame shows the statistically significant increases when the subject was silently carrying out *sequential subtractions* of 3 from 50, the thinking procedure being 50 → 47 → 44 → 41 → 38 etc., continuing on below 2 to − 1 → − 4 etc., until after the end of the recording of the rCBF at about 45 sec. During this whole period the subject was undisturbed by the environment. The first disturbance after the rCBF recording period was by the investigator who asked the subject the last number reached by the subtraction procedure. It is remarkable that the significantly increased rCBF's were on both sides in the prefrontal lobe except for the angular gyrus in the parietal lobe with increases of 20.3 and 14.7%. Correspondingly, the clinical condition of acalculia has been observed with bilateral destruction of the angular gyrus.

In *Fig.* 5 the "jingle" frame shows that the rCBF increases when the silent thinking was concentrated on a task of jumping mentally to every second word of a well-known Danish nonsense word sequence or jingle which consists of a closer loop of 9 words. Again almost all of the activated cortical areas were in the frontal lobe. The area of the right temporal lobe with a 16.5% increase was uniquely involved in jingle thinking and had previously been implicated in discrimination of auditory inputs[27].

The lowest frame of *Fig.* 5 gives the rCBF's during a route-finding paradigm, which is designed to test the effects of silently thinking sequential visual scenes. The subjects lying silently with eyes sealed had to imagine what they saw when they walked out of their front door into the street and turned left, then right at the next corner, left at the next and so on. It involved an immense amount of silent visual thinking, and correspondingly the cortical rCBF map was more complex bilaterally, and with the involvement of visual areas. Unfortunately the ^{133}Xe testing procedure gives little information from the occipital and inferior temporal lobes because the internal carotid artery is distributed very little to these areas.

Despite the extreme differences in the types of silent

thinking — number sequences, word sequences, and visual sequences — *Fig. 5* shows that in all three there was activation of the same cortical areas of both hemispheres, particularly in the superior and mid-frontal lobes. The similarities and differences are shown in the superimposed cortical maps of *Fig. 6*. Notable in *Fig. 6* are the uniquely activated areas

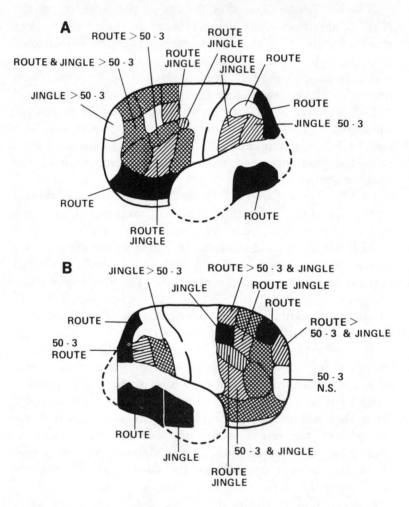

Fig. 6: *Diagram of differences in cortical activations during three different types of thinking. Areas that were specifically and statistically significantly activated in one type of thinking only are shown black. Areas activated by two types of thinking only are shown hatched. A: left hemisphere; B: right hemisphere (Roland and Friberg, 1985)*[25].

shown in black. For example the occipital superior and the posterior inferior-temporal on both sides are the visual areas for route-finding, and the right mid-temporal is an auditory area for the jingle. The prefrontal lobe is most complexly involved and will require a finer grain of discrimination for elucidation in detail. There is an important negative finding in *Fig. 6,* namely that all these three types of silent thinking fail to generate significant increases in rCBF's in any of the primary or secondary motor and sensory cortical areas delineated in *Fig. 2.*

A quite different type of silent thinking was investigated by Roland *et al.*[26] utilizing a sequential motor task, but with the same ^{133}Xe technique. In the initial investigation the subject continuously carried out a learned movement during the rCBF measurement. The particular example chosen was to touch rapidly the thumb by each finger in turn, two touches by finger 1, one by finger 2, 3 by finger 3 and 2 by finger 4, then reverse, 2 to 4, 3 tot 3, 1 to 2 and 2 to 1, and so on. The subject learns this motor sequence, as it is called, so that it is carried out without error, but it still requires concentrated thinking. In *Fig. 7A* the rCBF map shows large increases in the motor and sensory areas for fingers and thumb (cf. *Fig. 2)* on the contralateral side, which is in accord with the well-known crossed innervation of limbs by the cerebral cortex. But also in *Fig. 7A* there is activation of an area that is largely on the medial side of the frontal cortex, and this activation of the supplementary motor area (SMA), as it is called, is bilateral and just about as strong as for the motor cortex. The primary role of the SMA in voluntary movement is disclosed in *Fig. 7B.* With prior instruction and training the subject is able to carry out the motor sequence test by silent thinking in the absence of any movement, which is checked by continuous electromyographic recording. Under such conditions the SMA is bilaterally activated on both sides by the internal programming, as it is called, and there is no significant increase in rCBF in any other cortical area. *Fig. 7B* thus indicates a very selective action by silent thinking of a learned motor movement.

Fig. 7 illustrates an important caveat that enters into all

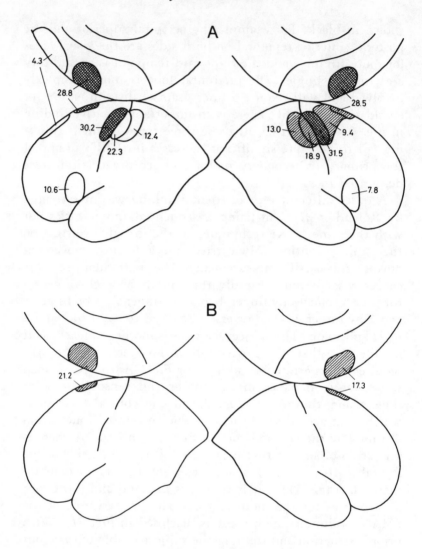

Fig. 7: A. *Mean increase of the rCBF in percent during the motor-sequence test performed with the contralateral hand, corrected for diffuse increase of the blood flow. Cross-hatched areas have an increase of rCBF significant at the 0.0005 level. Hatched areas have an increase of rCBF significant at the 0.005 level, for other areas shown the rCBF increase is significant at the level 0.05. Left: left hemisphere, five subjects. Right: right hemisphere, 10 subjects. B. Mean increase of rCBF in percent during internal programming of the motor-sequence test, values corrected for diffuse increase of the blood flow. Left: left hemisphere, three subjects; right: right hemisphere, five subjects (Roland et al., 1980)*[26].

the rCBF maps. Since the silent thinking of the motor sequence activates only the SMA *(Fig. 7B)*, it can be assumed that the additional activation with the motor sequence movements *(Fig. 7A)* is due to the excitatory action of the SMA neurons on the motor cortex. The further activation of the somatosensory area could be attributed to sensory feedback from the finger and thumb movement. Thus it is not necessary to assume that the thinking *directly* activated the areas in *Fig. 7A* additional to those in *Fig. 7B*. Similarly in *Fig. 5* many of the activated areas could be secondary to a few that are primarily activated. In the three types of silent thinking it could be that the primary action is on areas of the superior prefrontal cortex on both sides (cf. *Fig. 6)* and these in turn cause the activation of the other areas, but there is as yet no experimental evidence for this as there is in *Fig. 7*. Possibly the primary action of the silent thinking in *Fig. 4* is on the area of the mid-prefrontal cortex, which secondarily involves that area of the somatosensory cortex corresponding to the mental concentration.

3. THE BRAIN-MIND PROBLEM

The empirical findings illustrated in *Figs. 4, 5, 6* and 7 have great philosophical significance with respect to the brain-mind problem. The mental processes of silent thinking evoke remarkable responses in the brain and these responses exhibit a topography that is different for different types of thinking. It is important to recognize that the ^{133}Xe technique can give only a crude spatio-temporal pattern and that much of the activity may be due to subsequent neuronal activation; but this must not obscure the significance of the discovery that the mental events of silent thinking occur in conjunction with specific patterns of response in the cerebral cortex. It was surprising to find that the silent thinking for the jingle and route-finding procedures evoked increases in the total blood flow to the brain which were in excess of that occurring in intense perceptual and motor tasks[25]. There is good justification for the conclusion that silent thinking is hard brain work! It has been an invariable finding that in the deepest mental relaxation the frontal lobes retain a level of rCBF higher than any other areas of the cortex. Possibly this is generated by all the random thinking in the awake state, which is sometimes referred to as daydreaming[16].

In general terms there are two theories about the relationship of mental events to neural events.

Firstly, there is the explanation inherent in all monistic-materialisms, including all the varieties of parallelism, pan-psychism, epiphenomenalism and the now-fashionable iden-tity theory. The existence of mental events is not denied, but they are given a subsidiary role in the performance and experience of a human person, which is entirely brain con-trolled. For example, in the identity theory the mental events are somehow regarded as "identical" with neural events of a special kind in the highest levels of the brain, as succinctly expressed by Feigl[12]: "The identity thesis which I wish to clarify and to defend asserts that the states of direct experience which conscious human beings 'live through', and those which we confidently ascribe to some of the higher animals, are identical with certain (presumably configura-tional) aspects of the neural processes in those organisms ... processes in the central nervous system, perhaps especially in the cerebral cortex.... The neurophysiological concepts refer to complicated highly ramified patterns of neuron dischar-ges." (pp. 79 and 90)

As Popper[23] points out, all materialist theories of the mind "assert that the physical world (World 1) is self-con-tained or *closed....* This physicalist principle of the closed-ness of the physical World 1 is of decisive importance ... as the characteristic principle of physicalism or materialism" (p. 51).

Secondly, there is the dualist-interactionist explanation which has been specially developed for the self-conscious mind and human brain. It is proposed that superimposed upon the neural machinery in all its performance, there are at certain sites of the cerebral hemispheres (the so-called liaison areas) effective interactions with the self-conscious mind, both in receiving and in giving *(Fig. 8).*

4. A NEW HYPOTHESIS OF BRAIN-MIND INTERACTION

The materialist critics argue that insuperable difficulties are encountered by the hypothesis that immaterial mental events such as thinking can act in any way on material structures such as neurons of the cerebral cortex, as is diagrammed in *Fig. 8.* Such a presumed action is alleged to

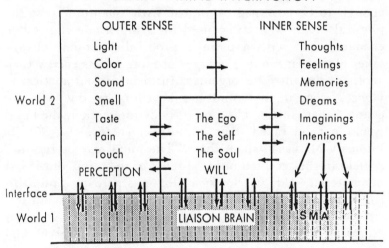

Fig. 8: *Information flow diagram for brain-mind interaction in human brain. The three components of World 2: outer sense; inner sense; and the psyche, self or soul; are diagrammed with their communications shown by arrows. Also shown are the lines of communication across the interface between World 1 and World 2, that is from the liaison brain to and from these World 2 components. The liaison brain has the columnar arrangement indicated by the vertical broken lines. It must be imagined that the area of the liaison brain is enormous, with open or active modules numbering over a million, not just the few here depicted. SMA: sensori-motor area.*

be incompatible with the conservation laws of physics, in particular of the first law of thermodynamics. This objection would certainly be sustained by 19th century physicists and by neuroscientists and philosophers who are still ideolo-

gically in the physics of the 19th century, not recognizing
the revolution wrought by quantum physicist in the 20th
century. Unfortunately it is rare for a quantum physicists to
dare to intrude into the brain-mind problem. But in a recent
book the quantum physicist Margenau[21] makes a fundamental contribution. It is a remarkable transformation
from 19th-century physics to be told, "that some fields,
such as the probability field of quantum mechanics carry
neither energy nor matter" (p. 22). He goes on to state:
"In very complicated physical systems such as the brain, the
neurons and sense organs, whose constituents are small
enough to be governed by probabilistic quantum laws, the
physical organ is always poised for a multitude of possible
changes, each with a definite probability; if one change
takes place that requires energy, or more or less energy than
another, the intricate organism furnishes it automatically.
Hence, even if the mind has anything to do with the
change, that is if there is a mind-body interaction, the mind
would not be called upon to furnish energy" (p. 96). In
summary Margenau states that: "The mind may be regarded
as field in the accepted physical sense of the term. But it is a
nonmaterial field, its closest analogue is perhaps a probability field. It cannot be compared with the simpler nonmaterial fields that require the presence of matter (e.g., gravity).
Nor does it necessarily have a definite position in space. And
so far as present evidence goes it is not an energy field in any
physical sense, nor is it required to contain energy in order
to account for all known phenomena in which mind interacts
with brain" (p. 97).

   In formulating more precisely the dualist hypothesis of
brain-mind interaction, the initial stament is that the whole
world of mental events (World 2) has an existence as autonomous as the world of matter-energy (World 1) *(Fig. 1)*.
The present interactionist hypothesis does not relate to these
ontological problems, but merely to the mode of action of
mental events on neural events, that is, of the nature of the
downward arrows across the frontier in *Fig. 8*. Following
Margenau[21] the hypothesis is that brain-mind interaction is
analogous to a probability field of quantum mechanics,
which has neither mass nor energy, yet can cause effective

action at microsites. More specifically it is proposed that the mental concentration involved in intentions *(Fig. 7)* or attention *(Fig. 4)* or planned thinking *(Figs. 5, 6)* can cause neural events by a process analogous to the probability fields of quantum mechanics.

We can ask: what neural events could be appropriate recipients for mental fields that are analogous to quantal probability fields? Already we may have the answer in recent discoveries on the nature of the synaptic mechanism whereby one nerve cell communicates with another.

Fig. 9A is a diagrammatic representation of a nerve cell of the cerebral cortex showing the soma with a long apical dendrite studded with spines on each of which there is a synapse from a nerve terminal derived from some other nerve cell. There are about 10,000 spine synapses on each pyramidal cell. *Fig. 9B* gives a diagram of such a synapse showing the nerve fiber expanded to a terminal bouton that makes a close contact with a special membrane thickening of the spine. In the bouton are numerous vesicles each of which contains 5,000 to 10,000 molecules of the specific synaptic transmitter substance, which is glutamate or aspartate for the great majority of excitatory boutons in the cerebral cortex. Some synaptic vesicles are in close contact with the presynaptic membrane confronting the postsynaptic membrane across the extremely narrow synaptic cleft. These synaptic vesicles appear to be arranged between dense projections.

Further structural analysis particularly by the freeze-fracture technique of Akert and associates[1,2] has led to the construction of a diagram of an idealized spine synapse *(Fig. 10)*, which is shown in perspective with partial excisions to reveal the deeper structures. The relatively loose arrangement of synaptic vesicles and presynaptic dense projections *(Fig. 9B)* is shown in *Fig. 10* as the precise packing illustrated in the inset on the left, with the synaptic vesicles in hexagonal array packaged between the presynaptic dense projections in triangular array. This composite structure is termed a presynaptic vesicular grid and it can be regarded as having paracrystalline properties[1,32]. The boutons of brain synapses have a single presynaptic vesicular grid, as is indicated in *Figs. 9B* and *10*.

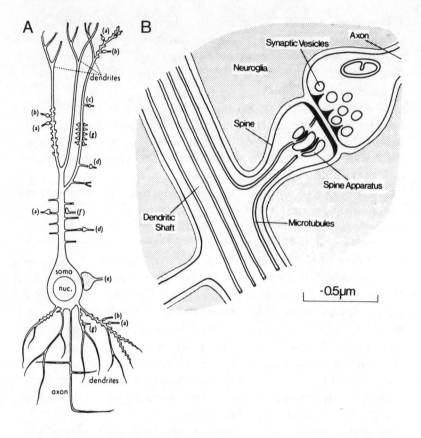

Fig. 9: *Synaptic endings on neurons. A. Drawing of a hippocampal pyramidal cell to illustrate the diversity of synaptic endings on the different zones of the
apical and basal dendrites, and the inhibitory synaptic endings on the soma.
The various types of synapses marked by the letters A to G are shown in higher
magnification to the right (Hamlyn, 1962)[14]. B. Drawing of a synapse on a
dendritic spine. The bouton contains synaptic vesicles and dense projections on the
presynaptic membrane (Gray, 1982)[13].*

There are only approximate figures for the number of
synaptic vesicles incorporated in a presynaptic vesicular
grid. The usual number appears to be 30 to 50 from the
illustrations of Akert et al.[1,2]. Thriller and Korn[32] give the
number as 44-83 for the boutons on Mauthner cells. Thus
only a very small proportion of the synaptic vesicles of a
bouton (about 20,000) are embedded in the firing zone of

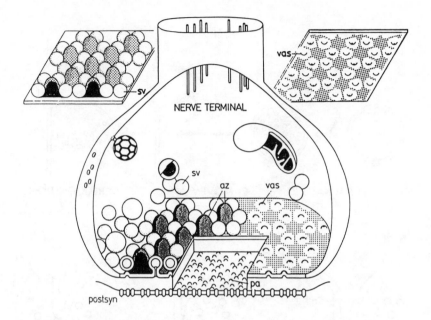

Fig. 10: *Schema of the mammalian central synapse. The active zone is formed by presynaptic dense projections (az). The postsynaptic aggregation of intra-membraneous particles is restricted to the area facing the active zone, sv = synaptic vesicles, pa = particle aggregations on postsynaptic membrane (post-syn.). Note synaptic vesicles (sv) in hexagonal array, as is well seen in the upper left inset, and the vesicle attachment sites (vas) in the right inset. Further description in text. (Akert et al., 1975)*[1]

the presynaptic vesicular grid. The remainder are loosely arranged in the interior of the bouton, as is partly shown in *Figs. 9B* and *10*.

Fig. 11A well illustrates the packaging of transmitter molecules into a synaptic vesicle and its movement up to the presynaptic vesicular grid by showing the presynaptic density of the presynaptic grid. Finally in *Fig. 11B* there is apposition to the presynaptic membrane under the influence of Ca^{2+} ions and the total release of the transmitter molecules into the synaptic cleft. The very close contact of the vesicle to the presynaptic membrane *(Fig. 11B2)* is also depicted in the left of *Fig. 10* with the two little bulges and one vesicle apparently ready to discharge, while to the right of *Fig. 10*, after the vesicles and the dense projections have

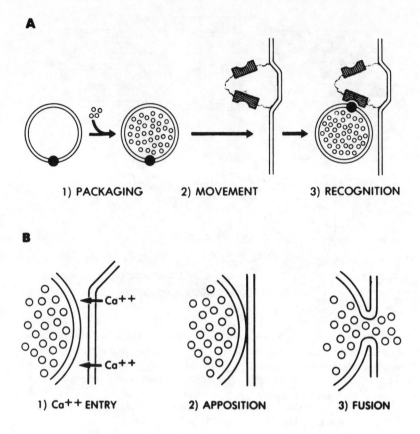

Fig. 11: *Stages of synaptic vesicle development, movement and exocytosis. A. The three steps involved in filling a vesicle with transmitter and bringing it to attachment to a presynaptic dense projection of triangular shape. B. Stages of exocytosis with release of transmitter into the synaptic cleft depicting the essential role of Ca^{2+} input from the synaptic cleft (Kelly et al., 1979)[18].*

been stripped off, the vesicle attachment sites *(vas)* are seen in hexagonal array, as also in the inset diagram to the right.

By precise analysis of the postsynaptic potentials generated when a presynaptic impulse activates a single bouton *(Fig. 9A, 10)*, it has been shown that the vesicular emission from a bouton (exocytosis) is probabilistic and below unity — the usual probability being 0.5 or less[17,19]. This probability can be varied up or down according to circumstances. The presynaptic vesicular grid must have some subtle func-

tional organization in controlling exocytosis of the embedded vesicles. It is proposed that mental events such as
intention *(Fig. 7)*, attention *(Fig. 4)* or silent thinking
*(Figs. 5, 6), change the probability of synaptic vesicular emission
in the manner suggested by Margenau* (pp. 96, 97)[21]. It is not
postulated that the firing of neurons is the target of the
mental events, but merely that this firing is modified by
alterations of the probabilities of quantal emission of those
synapses that are engaged in actively exciting them. This is
an important limitation in the target for events such as the
varieties of mental concentration in *Figs 4, 5, 6, 7*.

The *first question* that can be raised concerns the magnitude of the effect that could be produced by a probability
wave of quantum mechanics. Is the mass of the synaptic
vesicle so great that it lies outside the range of the uncertainty principle of Heisenberg? Margenau (p. 384)[20]
adapts the usual uncertainty equation for this calculation of
non-atomic situations:

$$\Delta x \, \Delta v \geq \frac{K}{M},$$

where $K = 1,06 \times 10^{-27}$ erg-sec, and the mass (M) of a
synaptic vesicle 40 nm in diameter can be calculated to be
10^{-18} g for example.

However, in *Fig. 11B* it can be seen that the mass criti-
cally involved in the exocytosis is much less than the mass of
a vesicle which is already in position (cf. *Figs 10, 11B2*). All
that is required is the displacement of a small area of the
double membrane. This area as depicted in *Figs 11B2* to
11B3 would be no more then 10 nm thick, and if it was
10 nm by 10 nm in area it would have a mass of only
10^{-18} g. If the uncertainty of the position, Δx, of the
contact site is taken to be 1 nm, then Δv, the uncertainty
of the velocity, is 10 nm in 0.1 msec, which is of the order
expected for the exocytotic opening seen in *Fig. 11B3*. Since
the vesicle is already in position *(Fig. 11B2)* in the presynaptic vesicular grid *(Fig. 10)*, the exocytosis is not dependent on movement through a viscous medium. The postulated mental influence would do no more than alter the
probability of emission of a vesicle already in apposition.

It can be concluded that calculations on the basis of the

Heisenberg uncertainty principle show that the probabilistic
emission of a vesicle from the presynaptic vesicular grid
could conceivably be modified by a mental intention acting
analogously to a quantal probability field.

The *second question* raises the order of magnitude of the
effect, which is merely a change in probability of emission of
a single vesicle *(Fig. 10, 11)*. This is many orders of magnitude too small for modifying the patterns of neuronal
activity even in small areas of the brain. However, there are
many thousands of similar boutons on a pyramidal cell of the
cerebral cortex *(Fig. 9A)*. The hypothesis is that the probability field of the mental intention is widely distributed not
only to the synapses on that neuron, but also to the synapses
of a multitude of other neurons with similar functions.

According to the microsite hypothesis, the presynaptic
vesicular grid provides *the chance* for the mental intention to
change *by choice* the probability of its synaptic emission. This
would be happening over the whole ensemble of spine synapses that are activated at that time, probably even
thousands, since there are about 10,000 on a single cortical
pyramidal cell[30]. It would be expected that a mental influence analogous to a probability field would exert a global
influence on the synapses of an appropriate neuron modifying up or down the probabilities of vesicular emission by
incoming impulses. So the *reliability* of mental intention is
derived from integration of the *chance happenings* at the multitude of presynaptic vesicular grids on that neuron.

As already mentioned, Margenau[24] makes the prescient
statement that in the postulated action of a mental event on
a neuronal event at microsites, there need be no energy
requirement: "If one change takes place that requires energy
... the intricate organism furnishes it automatically". Our
attention should be focussed on the exocytosis of a vesicle as
indicated in *Fig. 11B2* to *3*. Though the displacement of
the apposition membrane may require a minute energy, the
exocytotic release of the stored transmitter molecules in
Fig. 11B3 could be a source of energy. Thus on the microsite hypothesis the probability of exocytosis in response to a
nerve impulse may be altered by a mental event without an
energy requirement. The conservation laws would remain
inviolate.

5. TESTING OF BRAIN-MIND THEORIES

We can raise the question whether there could be experimental testing of predictions from the dualist-interactionist hypothesis *(Fig. 8)* on the one hand and the identity hypothesis on the other. A simple diagram *(Fig. 12A)* embodies the essential features of the identity hypothesis. In accord with Feigl[12] mental-neural identity occurs only for neurons or neuron systems at a high level of the brain, especially in the cerebral cortex. These neurons can be called mental-neural event (MNE) neurons, whereas other neurons in the brain, and in particular neurons on the input and output pathways, would be no more than simple neural event (NE) neurons, as in the diagram *(Fig. 12A)*. It would be predicted from the identity hypothesis that MNE neurons would be distinctive because in special circumstances their firing would be in unison with mental events. But of course this firing would be in response to inputs from other neurons, MNE or NE, and is in no way *determined* by or *modified* by the mental events. This is the *closedness of the physical world* referred to above[23].

However, the diagram of *Fig. 12A* is challenged by the evidence that internally generated thoughts strongly excite neurons in special areas of the cerebral cortex (Fig. 4, 5, 6, 7). These findings require the diagrammatic addition of an input from mental events (ME) *per se* as is shown by the additional arrows in the diagram *(Fig. 12B)*. The firing of MNE neurons would exhibit a response that is different from what it would be in the absence of the mental events of attention, silent thinking or intention as is shown in *Figs 4, 5, 6, 7. Fig. 12B* is a diagrammatic representation of dualist interactionism.

We can return to *Fig. 1* with the juxtaposed World 1 and World 2 each with a fundamental primacy, something that we have to accept as given, as two distinct orders of existence. In that context it can be appreciated that this lecture describes an attempt to show how microsites in the brain could have transcendental properties of being channels of communication between these two completely disparate existences. The philosophical implications could be far

54

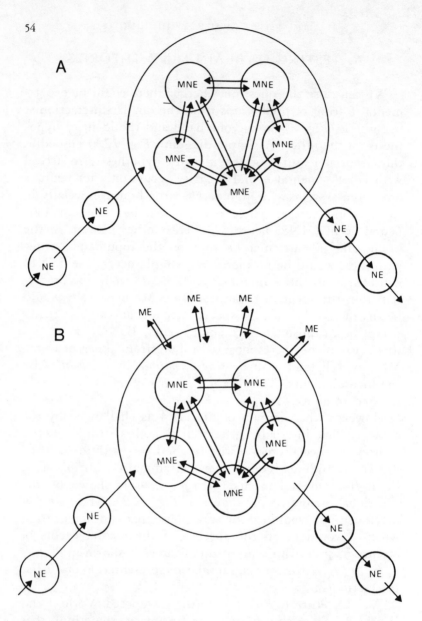

Fig. 12: *Diagrams of brain-mind theories. A. The identity theory. B. Dualist-interactionism. Assemblages of neurons are shown by circles. NE represents the conventional neurons which respond only to neutral events. MNE are neurons that are associated with both mental and neural events and are grouped in a larger circle representing the higher nervous system. In B, ME arrows represent mental influences acting on the neural population that is associated both with mental and neural events. All other arrows in A and B represent the ordinary lines of neural communication which are shown in reciprocal action.*

reaching if it comes to be accepted that mental events can effectively act on the brain as indiciated in *Figs 4, 5, 6, 7, 8*. We all think and act as if we have at least some control and responsibility for our actions, especially our linguistic expressions, but reductionist critics have insisted that this must be an illusion since it is contrary to the conservation laws of physics. We are now free to reject these criticisms.

It may seem beyond belief that the immense neuronal activity demonstrated in *Fig. 5* can be generated by internal thinking that initially merely modifies the probability of quantal emission from synaptic boutons. However, an essential component of the microsite hypothesis is that the mental event of thinking is widely distributed to the boutons of one pyramidal cell (cf. *Fig. 9A*) taking advantage of the design feature of an immense number of boutons ($\sim$ 10,000) on one such cell. Hence there is opportunity for great amplification at the primary site of action with the consequent bursts of impulse discharges such as was observed with SMA neurons in responses to voluntary movements of mokeys[5].

From the postulated net zero energy influence on the probability of vesicular emission at one microsite, there are three factors giving an immense amplification: the many microsites on one pyramidal cell; the many pyramidal cells subjected to the same mental influence — a functional cluster; the spreading excitation from the excited pyramidal cells by their axon collaterals and the excitatory stellate cells in the adjacent cortex. Hence we can account for the high level of "brain work" observed by Roland and Friberg[25].

On the microsite hypothesis it would be predicted that the interaction with mental events would be reduced to zero when the presynaptic firing background was reduced to zero. Lost of consciousness would occur, and be irreversible unless there would be revival to a considerable degree of the impulse discharges in the cerebral cortex. An example is "vigil coma" that supervenes when brain injury to the mid-brain turns off the reticular activating system[15,9]. In fact the principal role of the reticular activating system may be to provide a background of excitatory synaptic actions on neurons of the cerebral cortex with an immense array of

probabilistic vesicular emissions that are targets for the
quantal probabilistic fields of mental influences.

6. SUMMARY STATEMENTS ON THE BRAIN-MIND PROBLEM

A general observation is that hitherto all hypotheses attempt to give some explanation of how conscious experiences
derive from or relate to neural events in the active cerebral
cortex, as was done by Feigl[12]. Sperry[29] proposed that
mental events are holistic configurational properties of the
brain process. Mountcastle[22] developed the concept of distributed systems which are "composed of large numbers of
modular elements linked together in echeloned parallel and
serial arrangements", and are thought to provide an objective mechanism of conscious awareness. Edelman[11] suggested that "the brain processes sensory signals and its own
stored information upon this selective base in a phasic (cyclic) and re-entrant manner that is capable of generating the
necessary conditions for conscious states". Szentágothai[31]
suggested that "dynamic patterns" offer "superstructures"
and might be helpful to give a scientific explanation on the
higher functions of the brain including even consciousness.
Eccles[10] suggested that "the mental influence is exerted on
an extremely complex dynamic system of interacting
neurons".

The extreme alternative to these "nebular" hypotheses is
now proposed, namely that the essential locus of the action
of non-material mental events on the brain is at individual
microsites, the presynaptic vesicular grids of the boutons,
each of which operates in a probabilistic manner in the
release of a single vesicle in response to a presynaptic impulse. It is this probability that is assumed to be modified
by a mental influence acting analogously to a quantal probability field in the manner described above. The mechanism
by which effective action at microsites becomes amplified by
conventional neural circuitry will be dependent on the complex circuits envisioned, for example, by Feigl[12], Sperry[29],

Mountcastle[22], Edelman[11], Szentágothai[31] and Eccles[9,10]. *The microsite hypothesis* can be proposed as a tentative beginning of a scientific study of the reflective loop proposed by Creutzfeldt[6] as opening up the independent symbolic world of the mind, which is the World 2 of Popper and Eccles[23]. In contrast to the "nebular" hypotheses it offers a unique challenge to molecular neurobiology.

REFERENCES

1. AKERT, K., PEPER, K. and SANDRI, C. (1975). Structural Organization of Motor End Plate and Central Synapses. In: *Cholinergic Mechanisms,* P.G. WASER (ed.). New York: Raven Press, pp. 43-57.

2. AKERT, K., PFENNINGER, K., SANDRI, C. and MOOR, H. (1972). Freeze Etching and Cytochemistry of Vesicles and Membrane Complexes in Synapses of the Central Nervous System. In: *Structure and Function of Synapses,* G.P. PAPAS and D.F. PURPURA (eds.). New York: Raven Press, pp. 67-86.

3. ARMSTRONG, D.M. (1981). *The Nature of Mind.* Ithaca, N.Y.: Cornell Univ. Press.

4. BELOFF, J. (1962). *The Existence of Mind.* London: MacGibbon and Kee.

5. BRINKMAN, C. and PORTER, R. (1979). Supplementary Motor Area in the Monkey: Activity of Neurons during Performance of a Learned Motor Task. *J. Neurophysiol.* 42: 681-709.

6. CREUTZFELDT, O.D. (1979). Neurophysiological Mechanisms and Consciousness. In: *Brain and Mind,* CIBA Foundation Series 69. Amsterdam: Elsevier-North Holland, pp. 217-233.

7. DENNETT, D.C. (1969). *Content and Consciousness.* New York: Humanities Press.

8. DESMEDT, J.E. and ROBERTSON, D. (1977). Differential Enhancement of Early and Late Components of the Cerebral Somatosensory Evoked Potentials during Forces-Paced Cognitive Tasks in Man. *J. Physiol.* 271: 761-782.

9. ECCLES, J.C. (1980). *The Human Psyche.* Berlin-Heidelberg-New York: Springer.

10. ECCLES, J.C. (1980). How the Self Acts on the Brain. *Psychoneuroendocrinology* 7: 271-283.

11. EDELMAN, G.M. (1978). Group Selection and Phasic Reentrant Signalling: A Theory of Higher Brain Function. In: *The Mindful Brain,* Cambridge, Mass.: MIT Press pp. 51-100.

12. FEIGL, H. (1967). *The "Mental" and the "Physical".* Minneapolis, Minn.: University of Minnesota Press.

13. GRAY, E.G. (1982). Rehabilitating the Dendritic Spine. *Trends in Neurosciences* 5: 5-6.

14. HAMLYN, L.H. (1962). An Electron Microscope Study of Pyramidal Neurons in the Ammon's Horn of the Rabbit. *J. Anat.* 97: 189-201.

15. HASSLER, R. (1978). Interaction of Reticular Activating System for Vigilance and the Truncothalamic and Pallidal Systems for Directing Awareness and Attention under Striatal Control. In: *Cerebral Correlates of Conscious Experience.* P.A. BUSER and A. ROUGEUL-BUSER (eds.). Amsterdam: Elsevier-North Holland, pp. 110-129.

16. INGVAR, D.H. (1985). "Memory of the Future". An Essay on the Temporal Organization of Conscious Awareness. *Human Neurobiology* 4: 127-136.
17. JACK, J.J.B., REDMAN, S.J. and WONG, K. (1981). The Components of Synaptic Potentials Evoked in Cat Spinal Moto-neurons by Impulses in Single Group IA Afferents. *J. Physiol.* 321: 65-96.
18. KELLY, R.B., DEUTSCH, J.W., CARLSON, S.S. and WAGNER, J.A. (1979). Biochemistry of Neurotransmitter Release. *Ann. Rev. Neurosci.* 2: 399-446.
19. KORN, H. and FABER, D.S. (1986). Regulation and Significance of Probabilistic Release Mechanisms at Central Synapses. In: *New Insights into Synaptic Function,* G.M. EDELMAN, W.E. GALL and W.M. COWAN (eds.). New York: Neurosciences Research Foundation Inc., J. Wiley & Sons Inc.
20. MARGENAU, H. (1977). *The Nature of Physical Reality.* Woodbridge, Conn.: Ox Bow Press.
21. MARGENAU, H. (1984). *The Miracle of Existence.* Woodbridge, Conn.: Ox Bow Press.
22. MOUNTCASTLE, V.B. (1978). An Organizing Principle for Cerebral Function: The Unit Modul and the Distributed System. In: *The Mindful Brain,* pp. 7-50. Cambridge, Mass.: MIT Press.
23. POPPER, K.R. and ECCLES, J.C. (1977). *The Self and Its Brain.* Berlin-Heidelberg-New York: Springer.
24. ROLAND, P.E. (1981). Somatotopical Tuning of Postcentral Gyrus during Focal Attention in Man: A Regional Cerebral Blood Flow Study. *J. Neurophysiol.* 46: 744-754.
25. ROLAND, P.E. and FRIBERG, L. (1985). Localization in Cortical Areas Activated by Thinking. *J. Neurophysiol.* 53: 1219-1243.
26. ROLAND, P.E., LARSEN, B., LASSEN, N.A. and SKINOJ, E. (1980). Supplementary Motor Area and Other Cortical Areas in Organization of Voluntary Movements in Man. *J. Neurophysiol.* 43: 118-136.
27. ROLAND, P.E., SKINOJ, E. and LASSEN, N.A. (1981). Focal Activation of Human Cerebral Cortex during Auditory Discrimination. *J. Neurophysiol.* 45: 11139-1151.
28. RYLE, G. (1949). *The Concept of Mind.* London: Hutchinson.
29. SPERRY, R.W. (1976). Mental Phenomena as Causal Determinants in Brain Function. In: *Consciousness of the Brain,* G.G. GLOBUS, G. MAXWELL and I. SAVONDIK (eds.). New York: Plenum, pp. 163-177.
30. SZENTÁGOTHAI, J. (1978a). The Neuron Network of the Cerebral Cortex: A Functional Interpretation. *Proc. Roy. Soc. Lond.* B 201: 219-248.

31. SZENTÁGOTHAI, J. (1978b). The Local Neuronal Apparatus of the Cerebral Cortex. In: *Cerebral Correlates of Conscious Experience,* P. BUSER and A. ROUGEUL-BUSER (eds.). Amsterdam: Elsevier-North Holland, pp. 131-138.

32. TRILLER, A. and KORN, H. (1982). Transmission at a Central Inhibitory Synapse. III. Ultrastructure of Physiologically Identified and Stained Terminals. *J. Neurophysiol.* 48: 708-736.

THE BRAIN-MIND RELATIONSHIP

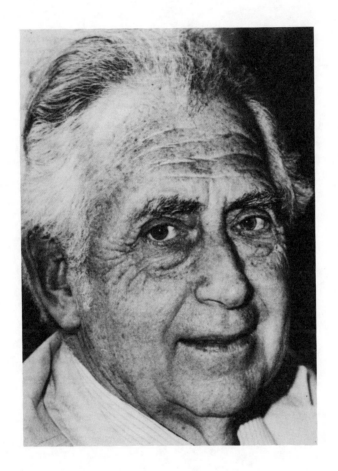

JÁNOS SZENTÁGOTHAI,

Emeritus Professor,
Semmelweis University Medical School,
First Department of Anatomy,
H 1450 Budapest, Hungary

INTRODUCTION

In view of my "Weltanschauung" — being a Christian believer, an active Protestant, brought up in the non-conformist tradition, now affiliated with the Lutheran Church — I would rather keep distanced from the philosophical side of the discussion. This attitude is strengthened by my lack of formal training in philosophy: my schooling as an adolescent suffered from a virtually complete "scotoma" in this field and later when — under other conditions — I might have tried to correct the shortcomings of my education, my circumstances for more than forty years did not create motivation for such an enterprize. Therefore, I remained a naive skeptic. First of all, I do not think that with today's understanding of matter, energy, and information, ancient concepts like "materialism versus idealism" or "monism versus dualism" make much sense — certainly not for me. These concepts seem to me hopelessly outdated, irrespective of any credo about the ultimate questions.

At the same time, being a scientist (or fancying myself so) I believe in the power and responsibility of reason. Since the Creator of the Universe (in my creed) is in no need of a "proof of existence", nor has to fear any "proof of non-existence", all questions are open to inquiry, and scientific studies should not be restricted by whatever ancient and venerable (although all too human), often metaphorical statements through which men of earlier periods could understand the ultimate questions of existence. But scientific inquiry is better off if it abides by two supreme laws: parsimony (the simplest possible explanation is almost always the best) and humility (nobody is entitled to think himself in sole possession of truth).

Fortunately, Otto Creutzfeldt, who in the good German tradition has done his homework in good time, has made it very clear on various occasions that if consciousness is taken as a reality, we have to accept some kind of duality, practically by definition. However, if I understand him correctly, this duality is not a dualism in the sense of Descartes, i.e., not a duality — or more exactly dualism — of substance (*rerum: res extensa* and *res cogitans*), but something else (I would again refrain from attaching any label, like "category" or anything you like). If such a view is at least philosophically tenable and cannot be proven absurd, out of hand I am well satisfied to leave things at this point.

As a neurobiologist who struggled for a lifetime with problems of the "blueprint" of the nervous system (the term meant in the narrowest sense of the word, i.e., connectivity of neurons), but as one who always tried to see the meaning behind the blueprint, I had to face thorny questions already at the very beginning of my studies. These questions arose mainly from aspects of "wholeness" versus "parts". It was already in my studies with the labyrinthine reflexes of eye and neck muscles that, beyond an unbelievable elegance and beauty of logic in the details, something was looming in the background that was more than the sum of the details. But this is quite trivial; C.S. Sherrington had understood and asked these questions explicitly well before I was born. The current discussion about the relationship between brain and mind is little else than the formulation of the age-old question at the contemporary level of the neurosciences.

I do not believe that I could significantly contribute to this discussion, apart from some basic "building blocks" or, to express it with more modesty, some pieces of the "jigsaw puzzle" that we are trying to put together; while being conscious that what is available to us is probably a tiny fraction of the total. I shall try to assemble my arguments around three such blocks: 1. *self-organization in neuronal nets;* 2. *the architectural principles upon which the assembly of neurons is based* (with some thoughts given to more general rules in connectivity of centers on the large scale); 3. *informational aspects of neural organization.*

1. SELF-ORGANIZATION IN NEURONAL NETWORKS

This part of the story has been told repeatedly — although generally rather cursorily — so that it might be summarized in the shortest possible way as follows. What should be stressed, though, is that for me subjectively, the central idea did not arise from my modern theoretical approach, but has arisen over many years of naive thinking about phenomena that my coworkers and I have observed. It was only much later that the convergence between our "nerve center recombination" techniques and modern theories of self-organization was realized.

It was during the late forties that we were playing at the Anatomy Department of Pécs University with my pupil György Székely with experiments on spinal cord regeneration. (In fact, I did such experiments early in 1938-39, when I observed the regenerative capacity of central neurons if brought into contact with degenerated peripheral nerves, i.e., empty Schwann cell tubes, but since it was always only very few fibers that did regenerate, I abondoned the subject. As we know now — although some naive students of the field still do not realize the simple fact — only mono-aminergic fibers have the capacity to regenerate at longer distances). Using newts *(Urodela; Triturus cristatus)* with the hope that these animals had a larger capacity for regeneration, we observed that after midthoracic transection of the spinal cord, the hindlimbs produced walking movements out of phase with the forelimbs. It was immediately obvious that this was the result of an external chain reflex, elicited by the friction of the belly on the surface when the forelimbs moved the animal. This phenomenon was known long ago, but we observed additionally that walking movements of the hindlimbs occurred only when the tail was distorted by contracture of its muscles. If the contracture was removed by gentle massage of the tail, the hindlimb reflex immediately subsided. This is again quite trivial: it was well known to earlier researchers that some minimal, although non-specific, input is needed — besides the specific sensory input (dragging of the belly skin over the surface) — to elicit the basic functional patterns of the isolated spinal cord. In accord with my romantic dispositions, I phrased the question as follows: "What causes the isolated lower half of the spinal cord to twist the tail in order to raise its non-specific sensory input?" The normal response, of course, would be: "ridiculous question, it is the over-excitability of neurons deprived of their normal input"! However, in this case the story is too good to be true. (Needless to say, in the then-prevailing atmosphere in Eastern Europe my timid attempt to communicate such thoughts — even only orally — met with an immediate outcry of indignation from the establishment).

Later more properly designed experiments were made[22] to test the questions (illustrated in *Fig. 1*): (a) what are the requirements for nerve cell assemblies to produce some regular — although biologically meaningless — output? Using the deplantation technique of Paul Weiss we soon found the answer:

(i) few mutually interconnected excitatory and inhibitory interneurons could produce repetitive sequences of bursts of activity; no organoid structure was required;

(ii) in our experimental situation motorneurons were needed because we used muscles as indicators; in tissue culture experiments, when one records directly, no motorneurons are needed;

(iii) no sensory input is necessary.

Fig. 1: *Tissue recombination experiments with isolated neural centers. Arrangement at left margin, showing the deplantation of neural centers and limb primordia into the dorsal fin of* Triturus *embryos. The drawing shows the situation in late larval stadia, when observations were made. A: Experiment of Székely and Szentágothai[22] described in the text. The deplanted center consists of few (15-25) scattered nerve cells, the motoneurons, which innervate the muscles of the implanted limb. Although the cells are mixed in reality, the motoneurons have been separated in the diagram because they served only as indicators. The generator of activity is shown at left as a randomly interconnected network of excitatory (outlines) and inhibitory interneurons (black). All of them connect also with the motoneurons serving as the output line of the interneuron network. B: Experimental arrangement of Székely and Czéh[23] where the deplanted center is a segment of the medullary tube ventral horn. If taken from the limb-bearing segments of the medullary tube, the innervated limb graft exhibits the cyclic "walking-type" movements of the limb illustrated by the circularly arranged heavy arrows; starting from the left "lift limb", "pull forward", "press down", and "push back". Further explanation in the text. C: The "parasitic" trunk-segment preparation of Brändle and Székely[1] illustrating the simple fact that the isolated limb segments of the medullary tube can move a pair of limbs only in parallel oarstroke-like manner; for the characteristic alternating movement pattern an additional part of the medullary tube, rostral from the limb segments, is necessary.*

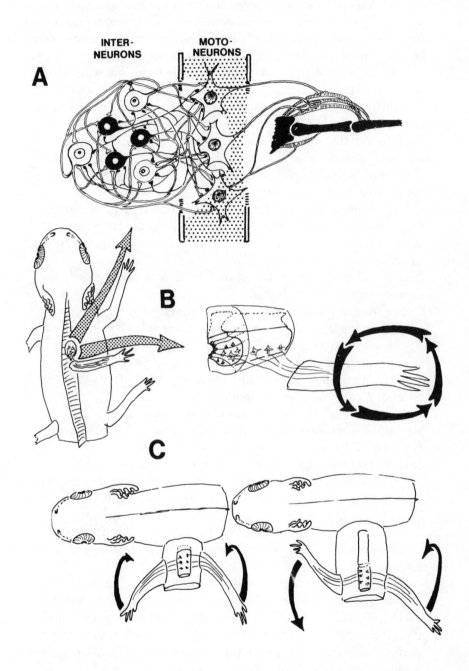

A

INTER-
NEURONS

MOTO-
NEURONS

B

C

Although we did not make such statements explicitly, we assumed that spontaneous random activity of the deplanted neurons became organized into the observed bursts of movement of the deplanted indicator limb.

Still later, Székely and Czéh[23] studied the question (b): what are the requirements of movements in essentially "walking patterns" produced by isolated spinal cord fragments and limbs? Using the same deplantation technique they found the simple answer:

(i) the segments of medullary tube had to come from "limb-segments" that are "designed" for this purpose; "non-limb" segments were ineffective;

(ii) the ventral half of the medullary tube had to retain its organoid structure, indicated by the presence of a central canal, the cells of which are the genetic matrix of spinal cord neurons;

(iii) the dorsal half of the spinal cord was not needed; no sensory input was required.

Eventually Brändle and Székely[1] analyzed the question of alternating step movements. Using a somewhat different "parasitic trunk segment" preparation, they found (c) that:

(i) one (or several [2-3] successive) segment(s) of the early isolated medullary tube could move a pair of limbs only in parallel "oarstroke" type movement;

(ii) for the natural alternating movement of any pair of limbs the preservation of a few additional segments rostral from the limb moving segments was required;

(iii) whether sensory input was required in such cases is not yet known for certain (due to limitations of this experiment) but from circumstantial evidence one may safely conclude that it was not!

It would be a distortion of the facts to claim that the significance of these observations was understood and interpreted explicitly at that time.

My conclusion today is: spontaneous random activity occurring in interconnected interneurons of medullary tube origin — i.e., "noise" in terms of information theory and engineering — is organized into an entirely unpredictable pattern of bursts of activity (in experiment "a"). Although meaningless biologically, this is "self-organization" because each individual preparation has its own distinctive overall repetitive (cyclic) pattern; i.e., the same bursts of activity reappear with very wide variations, but still within set limits. The "limits" are also, of course, set in this preparation also by which muscles of the limb receive their innervation by the few motorneurons. Since there is no feedback (of any known sort) either from motorneurons or from muscles to the "generator center", motorneurons can have no causal role. The experimental series under (b) shows that such "self-organized" activity can produce the characteristic output patterns of the medullary tube segment, provided that the excitatory and inhibitory interneurons are interconnected in the genetically predetermined patterns of connectivity, which is specific for the different parts of the spinal cord. The series under (c) shows that for the normal alternating stepping of a limb pair some additional "step alternation generator" is needed that is localized rostrally from the limb segments. Brändle and Székely[1] assumed that this might be part of the very ancient sinusoid vertebral column movement (swimming) of the vertebrates, but analogous experiments in birds[19,23] as well as some other embryonic recombination experiments[20,21] are more suggestive of some "holistic" (cooperative) element present even in the lower parts of the CNS.

For the purpose of the argument (and approach) presented here it fully suffices to assume that random spontaneous activity — known to exist in isolated neurons — is "self-organized" into various types of outputs, and that organized connectivity is not needed for the maintenance of cyclic activity. Organized connectivity is necessary, though, for higher levels of organized output.

2. PRINCIPLES OF NEURON NETWORK ARCHITECTURE AND SOME GENERALITIES ON CONNECTIVITY

The organization of neuron networks in assemblies of repetitive internal structure has been discussed in much detail over the last fifteen years. These repetitive units are generally referred to as "modules" and the organization of various centers according to this principle is called "modular organization". The idea of "neuron assemblies" was proposed first by Hebb[5], albeit with an entirely different objective. As a structural principle the roots go back (implicitly) to many of the early drawings of Ramón y Cajal[16,17]; and an explicit formulation of the structural principle was given first by M.A. and A.B. Schneibel[18]. After a vague attempt to formulate the concept in structural-functional terms[26] the concept was defined explicitly in the 1970s[27,28]. For the cerebral cortex this organization principle was forecast by earlier findings as an empirical, physiological unit under the name *columnar organization*[7,14].

Fig. 2 tries to give a radically simplified view of the

Fig. 2: *Architectural principle of the cerebral cortex. Upper part of the diagram shows that the cortex can be envisaged as a mosaic of vertical columns, defined by the convergence of a group of cortico-cortical afferents. Only pyramidal cells are illustrated from which those situated in the outer three layers of the cortex project exclusively to other parts of the cortex, where the fibres terminate as cortico-cortical afferents. Pyramid cells of the lower two layers project mainly to subcortical targets, but their collaterals, or some of the main branches, reach the cortex of the opposite hemisphere. Lower part of the diagram gives a radically simplified diagram of the cortical column: a vertical cylinder containing about 5,000 nerve cells, ∿ 60% pyramidal (Py, projective = output cells), ∿ 40% are interneurons of various kinds, 20% of the total are now known to be inhibitory. The cylindric column is defined anatomically by the cortico-cortical afferents (cortico-cortic.) placed into the axis of the cylinder. The specific sensory afferents (sens. aff.) are dominant only in the primary sensory areas, but secondary and further sensory areas have a similar input into lamina IV (lamination in Roman numerals at left margin) from the primary areas. The further local transmission of the specific input is indicated only by arrows (in outline if excitatory, and black if inhibitory). Two rows of large basket cells (Ba) at the border of layers III-IV and IV-V exercise inhibition over distances of up to 2-3 mm. This horizontal inhibition is assumed to narrow down the "waist" of the column in layers III-V (dark horizontal arrows), while excitation is conjectured to spread in radial direction both in lamina I and VI, either by the long terminal branches of cortico-cortical afferents in lamina I and pyramidal cell collaterals both in lamina I and VI. This distorts the original cylinder dynamically into the shape of an hourglass. The rich mutual local inhibitory and/or disinhibitory interconnections, oriented primarily in vertical direction, are not included in this diagram.*

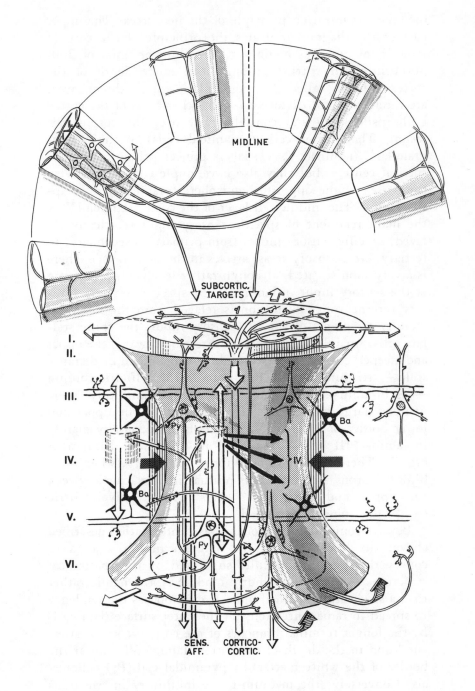

modular organization principle of the neocortex. The upper part of the diagram indicates the principle of the cortical moduls, assumed as being vertical columnar units of 200-300 μm width cutting through the entire depth of the cortex. The so called "supragranular" (outer three) layers are interconnected exclusively with other areas of the cortex both ipsilaterally and contralaterally over the corpus callosum. The output cells (pyramidal cells) of the "infra-granular" (laminae V, VI) layers project primarily to sub-cortical centers, but they also have ample connections with the cortex of the opposite hemisphere (practically none ipsilaterally). The middle cell layer of the cortex (lamina IV) is the main recipient of specific sensory input (cortically re-layed, specific sensory input, from primary to secondary, to tertiary, etc., sensory areas, arrives in the same layer). There is a very sophisticated, although rather localized, processing of the sensory input in lamina IV by specific sets of inhibi-tory interneurons. Excitation is relayed from the main ex-citatory recipients of specific sensory input (the spiny stel-late cells), mainly in the vertical direction towards the upper and deeper cortical layers. Inhibition on medium distance scale — reaching beyond the limits of the cylindric column — is brought about by two sets of large inhibitory inter-neurons (large basket cells (Ba) localized at the upper and lower border of Lamina IV, but acting horizontally mainly in laminae III and V indicated in the lower diagram of Fig. 2). There is an inhibitory (or disinhibitory, when inhi-bitory neurons are contacted) mutual interrelation between the upper and lower cell layers with relatively little (∿ 50 μm) tangential spread.

Beyond conveying some of the basic information described above, the lower part of the diagram in Fig. 2 tries to convey the idea — forcefully suggested by the anatomical structure — that the cylindric module is a dynamic rather than a structurally defined unit. Excitation has the tendency to spread in radial directions on the outer surface (lamina I) by the longer terminal branches of the cortico-cortical affer-ents[4] and in the depth of the cortex (lamina VI, and at the border of the white matter) by pyramidal cell (Py) collater-als. Conversely, the medium-range inhibitory interneurons in lamina IV, and the larger basket cells bordering lamina IV, limit the tangential spread of the excitation and are "corsetting the waist" of the columnar module. The shape of the column can, hence, be envisaged as a hyperboloid torus (hourglass) kept in dynamically changing fluctuation. Obviously, the column should not be understood as a single unit: from the $\sim$ 5,000 neurons of a column, the actual input can select smaller groups of active neurons (in the order of the tens), while other sets may be suppressed. Each pyramidal cell has a very powerful, specific inhibitory mechanism acting upon the initial part of the axon. These are the newly discovered "axo-axonic" or earlier "chandelier" cells.

Connectivity. There is a continuous connectivity at the range of about 10 neighbouring columns — in all possible directions — both excitatory over pyramid cell collaterals and inhibitory over the large basket cells. In the longer range, connectivity between different parts of the cortex is extremely rich, although very well addressed, probably almost exclusively by genetic factors. (Function, mainly in the cortical maturation period — postnatally in the human — may certainly contribute to addressing on the microscopic scale, but little, if at all, on the macroscopic pathway scale.) Over 80% of all output connections of the cortex are directly addressed to other regions of the cortex. The vast majority of all other efferent connections enter into loops over the upper brainstem nuclei, lower brainstem nuclei, and further over the cerebellum, which are in large part again readdressed to the cerebral cortex. Eventually the whole output of the CNS is monitored over the sensory system, so that all other activity of the brain is arranged over the outer world by an immensely complex system of external loops.

The net result of this makes one realize the most general principle of neural organization: *reentrance*. Reentrance is probably highest in the neocortex itself. (But this is not restricted to the cerebral cortex: although not so obvious, the same principle applies also to the cerebellum, for which this concept has been elaborated recently in the "cortico-nuclear microzone" concept of M. Ito[8], and it is probably

valid in most other major neutral centers). Quantitatively,
though not in complexity, reentrance is reduced in the
internal cerebral loop system, and reduced still further in
number, but becomes more complex in function in the outer
(external world) loop system. So our final conclusion has to
be that the nervous system is — or at least looks from the
structural side — much more a "self-contained" or "self-
reference" system, which is anchored in the external world
with many fewer channels of output to, and of input from,
the outside. It is, of course, arbitrary to label as "few" a
couple of million motorneurons and vegetative efferent
neurons and, say, ten times as many sensory channels. However, if compared to the total number of fifty billion neurons
(5×10^{10}) in the human nervous system, this is few indeed.

3. INFORMATIONAL ASPECTS OF NEURAL ORGANIZATIONS

I would agree with Otto Creutzfeldt's criticism of indis-
criminate use of Shannonian measures of information. These
measures are rendered almost meaningless by the ability of
the human nervous system (or mind, rather) to deal with
abstract symbols as well as, or better than, raw sensory
input. Nevertheless, information flow aspects of "neural"
or "mind" functions are still important. Donald M. Mac-
Kay has dealt with various aspects of this problem in an
impressive series of publications from 1951 onward. It is
frustrating to see how "legitimate neuroscience" and even
"mind-science" makes so little use of the impressive and
highly instructive information flow diagrams of Mac-
Kay[9,10,11,12,13].

> (My own personal experience with this field is that sometime
> around 1956[24] we tried to refute the generalized formula of v.
> Holst[6] on a so-called "reafference principle" of the nervous sys-
> tem on the basis of our "reversed-eye-transplantation" experi-
> ments. At the time, I had never heared of MacKay — due to my
> complete isolation and the limitations of journal subscription

outside my immediate fields of interest. It was more difficult to refute the similar — although ingeniously non-committally phrased — "corollary discharge" concepts of R.W. Sperry and H.L. Teuber. We were, of course, rather naive in our explanations, but our argument did correspond exactly to what MacKay could express with such superb clarity.)

It would be tantamount to courting disaster if I went into any details of the informational aspects. But one side of the problem cannot be neglected: all the speakers of today agree on the concept of *downward causation*, i.e., that whatever is in our mind or our consciousness can causally interfere with the physiological operations of our brain neuron circuits. For reductionists of any brand this is pure nonsense. But the real questin is how one is to envisage such an interference in the framework of the laws of thermodynamics, or in other words the widely held belief — which I do most emphatically share — in the closeness of nature. Sir John Eccles offers an explanation on the basis of the Heisenberg uncertainty principle.

I do think, though, that we do not really need to resort to such an *ultima ratio*.

Although this is still very controversial, many theorists in the fields of thermodynamics and "dynamic systems" are inclined to believe that there is some genuine and not purely formal relation between order (= negentropy) and information. Brillouin's[2] "negentropy principle of information" — although it would be a magnificent solution — is not accepted by the majority of theorists. My coworker, Péter Érdi[3], found an elegant solution by developing the conjecture illustrated in *Fig. 3,* based on recognizing the fallacy of a rigid separation of thermodynamic and information-theoretic entropy into two different categories; the first as if it were bound to, and the second as if it were entirely independent from physical reality. No information flow, one ought to realize — although this question is usually not raised in physics — is entirely free from the flow of energy and/or matter. Information flow can, therefore, be considered as a special "form" of matter and energy flow. A relationship between thermodynamic entropy and a *precisely determined* information-theoretic entropy can be assumed when,

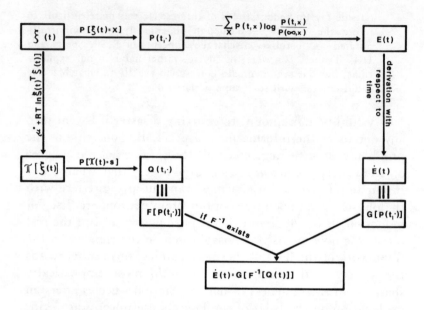

Fig. 3: *Derivation — by Péter Érdi*[3] *— of the relationship between the thermodynamic and information-theoretic entropy change.* Π *denotes the thermodynamic entropy production, considered as a stochastic process. Q is the distribution of* Π*, E is the Kullback-Rényi entropy with negative sign. Further explanation in the text.*

in a macroscopic stochastic system, the relation is symbolized as in *Fig. 3.* If considered as a stochastic process the value of the thermodynamic entropy Π is uniquely determined by the actual state of the system. The information-theoretic entropy E is determined by (the distribution of) *all possible* states, although not by the actual state itself. The Q distribution function of Π (i.e., the thermodynamic entropy production) and E (the information-theoretical entropy production) are the (generalized) functionals of the *same* function (P[t,·] i.e., the absolute distribution of the original process).

Accepting this solution, a "downward causal" relation between *information* (of what is in the mind) and what occurs in the neuron networks of the brain cannot be regarded as being outside or in contradiction to the basic laws of nature. Expressed in simpler words, dynamic activity patterns of neural networks, which we have tried to show exist as the result of the self-organization of random spontaneous activity in individual neurons, are *open to information*. This does not apply, obviously, to simple deterministic functions of neural chains, for example the "knee jerk"; but it will probably be very difficult to find the exact border between simple deterministic functions of neuronal chains and the point where "self-organization" comes in. However, in order to make some sense of the bits and pieces so far told, we have to try to put them together.

4. AN ATTEMPT TO JOIN SOME OF THE PIECES TOGETHER

In this view the nervous system is not a reflex robot (nor is it in the "preneural" organization of prokaryotic organisms like bacteria, nor in eukaryotes like protozoa) even in the simplest living forms. It is a "self-referential", highly autonomous — higher than life *(per se)* — level of organization. Its main driving force, at least in higher animals, is the spontaneous activity of its elements (the neurons), which becomes "self-organized" into dynamic activity patterns, analogous to the so-called "dissipative structures" of Prigogine. (We do not have to worry about the energetic side, because life in itself is kept up at the cost of the environment, and since neurons are living matter, this aspect can be taken for granted). The dynamic activity "structures" that have come about by self-organization as suggested in 1. are assumed to be (a) open for natural sensory input, (b) genetically inbuilt, (c) acquired (memory type) information, and — most important of all in the human — (d) the whole symbolic World 3 of Popper and Eccles (language, metalanguage, myths, abstract concepts from the simplest symbols of naive identity to the most complex symbolic systems in mathematics and philosophy). Although this is only a metaphorical phraseology, all nervous systems contain some model of the outside world, irrespective of whether this model is implicit (as is likely the case in all animals) or explicit (as is likely the case in man). What we experience as some kind of consciousness is in animals the system of implicit models and in our own consciousness the explicit models embodied most clearly in speech. But this is not exclusively so, because deaf-mute persons and those who have lost their speech by brain damage may be clearly conscious (probably as much as are normal persons).

The massive, multiple, and continuously repeated reentrance is the structural substrate of the intricate intertwinement of all neural activities from the most elementary reflexes, over our continuous interaction with the environment, up to our most abstract inner life experienced as our "self".

However, one should not forget that the "self", so beautifully placed at the center of the whole issue by Popper and Eccles[15], does not and cannot even exist without other selves. An infant deprived of its natural communication with its fellow beings — as exemplified by old stories, but dramatically shown by the famous case in California — does not develop a self that could even be compared to lower animal "selves". The "self" and our entire consciousness is, hence, the result of communication — or let me be more specific, of community — between different human beings. And let us return here to the first sentence of my talk: Christianity is probably unique among the religions of the human species in its emphasis on community — both between fellow humans and between man and the ultimate cause and reason of existence — as the very basic condition of our existence as individuals.

REFERENCES

1. BRÄNDLE, K. and SZÉKELY, Gy. (1973). The Control of Alternating Coordination of Limb Pairs in the Newt (Triturus Vulgaris). *Brain Behaviour and Evolution* 8: 366-385.

2. BRILLOUIN, L. (1962). *Science and Information Theory.* 2nd ed. New York: Academic Press.

3. ÉRDI, P. (1983). Hierarchical Thermodynamic Approach to the Brain. *Int. J. of Neurosci.* 20: 193-216.

4. GOLDMAN, P.S. and NAUTA, W.J.H. (1977). Columnar Distribution of Cortico-Cortical Fibers in the Frontal Association, Limbic, and Motor Cortex of the Developing Rhesus Monkey. *Brain Res.* 122: 393-413.

5. HEBB, D.O. (1949). *The Organization of Behaviour.* New York: Wiley.

6. HOLST, E.v. and MITTELSTAEDT, H. (1950). Das Reafferenzprinzip. *Naturwissenschaften* 37: 464-476.

7. HUBEL, D.H. and WIESEL, T.N. (1959). Receptive Fields of Single Neurons in the Cat's Striate Cortex. *J. Physiol.* 148: 574-591.

8. ITO, M. (1984). *The Cerebellum and Neural Control.* New York: Raven Press.

9. MacKAY, D.M. (1951). Mindlike Behaviour in Artefacts. *British J. of Phil. Sci.* 2: 105-121.

10. MacKAY, D.M. (1956). Towards an Information-Flow Model of Human Behaviour. *British J. of Phil. Sci.* 47: 30-43.

11. MacKAY, D.M. (1966). Cerebral Organization and the Conscious Control of Action. In: *Brain and Conscious Experience,* J.C. ECCLES (ed.). Berlin-Heidelberg-New York: Springer.

12. MacKAY, D.M. (1978). Selves and Brains. *Neuroscience* 3: 599-606.

13. MacKAY, D.M. (1980). The Interdependence of Mind and Brain. *Neuroscience* 5: 1389-1391.

14. MOUNTCASTLE, V.B. (1957). Modalities and Topographic Properties of Single Neurons of Cat's Sensory Cortex. *J. Neurophysiol.* 20: 408-434.

15. POPPER, K.R. and ECCLES, J.C. (1977). *The Self and Its Brain.* Berlin-Heidelberg-New York: Springer.

16. RAMON Y CAJAL, S. (1909). *Histologie du système nerveux de l'homme et des vertebrés.* I. Maloine.

17. RAMON Y CAJAL, S. (1911). *Histologie du système nerveux de l'homme et des vertebrés.* II. Maloine.

18. SCHNEIBEL, M.E. and SCHEIBEL, A.B. (1958). Structural Substrates for Integrative Patterns in the Brain Stem Reticular Core. In: *Reticular Formation of the Brain.* JASTER, H.H., PROCTOR, L.D., KNIGHTON, R.S., NOSHAY, W.C. and OSTELLO, R.T. (eds.). Little Brown and Co, pp. 31-55.

19. STRAZNICKY, K. (1963). Function of Heterotopic Spinal Cord Segments Investigated in the Chick. *Acta Biol. Hung.* 14 (2): 145-155.
20. SZÉKELY, G. (1959). Functional Specificity of Cranial Sensory Neuroblasts in Urodela. *Acta Biol. Hung.* 10 (1): 107-116.
21. SZÉKELY, G. (1959). The Apparent "Corneal Specificity" of Sensory Neurons. *J. Embryol. Exp. Morph.* Vol. 7 (3): 375-379.
22. SZÉKELY, G. and SZENTÁGOTHAI, J. (1962). Experiment with "Model Nervous Systems". *Acta Biol. Acad. Sci. Hung.* 12: 253-269.
23. SZÉKELY, G. and CZÉH, G. (1971). Activity of Spinal Cord Fragments and Limbs Deplanted in the Dorsal Fin of Urodele Larvae. *Acta Physiol. Sci. Hung.* 40: 303-312.
24. SZENTÁGOTHAI, J. and SZÉKELY, G. (1955). Elementary Nervous Mechanisms Underlying Optokinetic Responses, Analyzed by Contralateral Eye Grafts in Urodele Larvae. *Acta Physiol. Acad. Sci. Hung.* 10 (1): 43-55.
25. SZENTÁGOTHAI, J. (1961). Specificity and Plasticity of Neural Structures and Functions. In: *Brain and Behavior.* Vol. 1. Proceedings of the First Conference. M.A.B. BRAZIER (ed.), Washington: American Inst. Biol. Sci.
26. SZENTÁGOTHAI, J. (1967). The Anatomy of Complex Integrative Units in the Nervous System. In: *Recent Developments in Neurobiology in Hungary I,* K. LISSÁK (ed.), pp. 9-45. Budapest: Akadémiai Kiadó.
27. SZENTÁGOTHAI, J. and ARBIB, M.A. (1974). Conceptual Models of Neural Organization. *Neurosciences Research Program Bulletin* 12: 313-510.
28. SZENTÁGOTHAI, J. (1975). The "Module Concept" in Cerebral Cortex Architecture. *Brain Res.* 95: 475-496.

DISCUSSION

B. Gulyás (Catholic University of Leuven)

Professor Szentágothai, yesterday we heard about the basic building blocks of your theory: the self-organizing principles in nature and in the central nervous system, the modular organization of the neocortex, and the application of both MacKay's "information flow theory" and Érdi's thermodynamic theory to the functioning of the nervous system. But you did not explain in great detail your ideas concerning the global neural functions, how they are embodied in their biological background, i.e., the neuronal functioning of the brain. You did not explain an idea you often used to refer to, the so-called backward or downward causation in the central nervous system, and other such problems. We know that you sometimes allude to emergent ideas. So let me ask you to what extent is your theory similar to or different from Bunge's "emergent materialist theory", in which the mental phenomena are regarded as emergent properties and not as emergent entities, or to Sperry's "emergent monism", in which all mental phenomena can be regarded as a holistic emergent entity, which emerges from and at the same time is rooted in its biological background, the brain?

J. Szentágothai

Yes, thank you very much Dr. Gulyás. I must admit that when writing the prefatory article for the 1984 issue of the *Annual Review of Neuroscience* under the title "Downward

Causation?"[21] I was somewhat overconfident about being able to come up within reasonable time with a coherent brain-mind theory of my own. I thought that the "building blocks" you were referring to, such as (1) self-organization in neural tissues, (2) spontaneous activity arising in neurons (random neural noise) as the main source of the raw material that is being self-organized, (3) the modular architectonics principle of neural centers, especially of the cerebral cortex, and (4) the "information flow" concepts of D.M. MacKay, would automatically lead to the emergence of such a theory. Érdi's thermodynamic argument (5) about some formally definable relation between thermodyanmic and information theoretic entropy was used simply to resolve the apparent contradiction between "downward causation" and the laws of thermodynamics, especially the second law. I might mention that J.-P. Changeux and coworkers[4] have recently used similar mental strategies in speaking of spontaneously generated pre-representations and their resonance with activities produced by other conventional types of input.

Having realized that my 1983 (and prior) expectations did not materialize, I wanted to keep away from philosphical questions, especially in front of Sir John Eccles and Otto Creutzfeldt, whose knowledge and understanding of the philosophical issues I consider vastly superior to my own rather humble insight. But if you are asking me specifically, I do not agree either with the Bunge's concept on an "emergent materialist theory" or with Sperry's "emergent monism", although my antagonism to the two has entirely different motivations.

In the first statement of his theory Bunge[3] puts forward three major points of his *fifth postulate:*

"(i) All mental states, events and processes are states of, or events and processes in, the central nervous systems of vertebrates;

(ii) these states, events and processes are emergent relative to those of the cellular components of the CNS;

(iii) the so-called psychophysical relations are interactions between different subsystems of the CNS, or between them and other components of the organism."

I can fully agree with the first two, but am completely

lost with the third. I understand the words, of course, but I cannot understand what they mean. This third point does not explain anything to me, or only says something that is known anyway: i.e., that various parts of the nervous system are intimately interconnected, and so the nervous system is interconnected with all parts of the body. But this does not reveal anything about "global functions of the brain" that I am inclined to call the "mind". If it is claimed that the nervous system includes the model of the outer world, and that other parts of the brain contain models of this model, that is acceptable to me, although nobody knows what this means in neurobiological terms. As mentioned in my lecture, I am at loss with the terms "materialism" or "monism" or "dualism" for that matter. What is "matter" for today's physicist and cosmologist? Does it have any of its conventionl connotations of the earlier centuries? I think not. All of these concepts seem to me hopelessly outdated. Why do we have to quarrel about them?

My trouble with Sperry's concept is just the other way round. I admire his courage in having brought back consciousness as an emergent property and an operative principle in behavioural functions[20]. But I would be reluctant to give up the concept of closeness of our world as reflected in the basic laws of physics, especially of thermodynamics. I believe that there is some "downward causation" from the emergent "consciousness" level toward the level of the "functioning of neurons" — ... but how? I think that D.M. MacKay in his discussion with Sperry has given the best possible answer, but it would be unnecessary to reiterate his argument here. Érdi's reasoning about the two kinds of entropy are only to support the reasoning of MacKay.

However, since "the proof of the pudding is in the tasting", and in order to come down to practical consequences of our understanding of the brain for ethics and value systems, let me become very provocative. It is a very common dilemma in modern medicine whether or not to keep somebody on life-supporting (breathing, etc.) gadgets. If the doctors have convinced themselves that most of the cerebral cortex has been irreversibly damaged (criteria for this still need discussion), the patient although physiologically alive, is no longer a person and the gadgets should be unplugged. I would wish this to be done with myself and with anybody close to my heart. Conversely, the same argument would be false if it concerned a human embryo. One might argue about — using some yet unavailable statistics — whether or not one should consider the embryo a human being as such from the moment of conception, or, say, six and one-half days later when implanted *in utero*. But it is immaterial whether there is any nervous system already, because in well over 90% of the cases the early neural tube will develop into a (normal) human brain.

So you see our views of brains and minds have very serious practical consequences.

J. Eccles

First of all, let me ask a question: when a subject is unconscious with an EEG of delta waves showing very low brain activity you want to know how long you go on before you take him off the machine? Every night when we go to sleep we are unconscious, but our brains are active. One has to think what is involved in this brain activity. It is too simplistic to say: "there is no brain activity, hence the mind doesn't exist or the soul doesn't exist". Even after months of deep vigil coma consciousness may return. We have to see how far we can understand the brain and mind interaction.

I was trying to give you yesterday a precise microsite story, which gets us down to something which is in part scientifically testable and understandable, and which is based on the latest discoveries. The microsite theory is the theory of how a mental event can change the probability of emission of vesicles in the synapses without breaking the conservation laws of physics. This was the statement I made and this is also Margenau's statement. Here is a vesicle (see *Figure 9* in my paper), here is the membrane, and you just open this minute gate and the contents move out. That is how it normally works, and all you are doing is altering the probability of the synaptic emission by the mental event and it works analogously to a probability wave of quantum mechanics.

The big question is: what is the nature of the mind? That is beyond answering. We have to take it as given, it is a reality. This is rejected by those who want to make the mind secondary, emerging from the brain. It is a reality apart from the brain as much as the brain is a material reality. They are two worlds, World 1 and World 2 of Popper and mine[18]. This is something we cannot explain, but we cannot explain matter either. Let's take gravitation, for example. We cannot explain gravitation. We have to live and work with entities which are beyond our understanding; we have to live with our experienced existence, our experienced uniqueness. The life we have is a mental life in the first place, the using of our brains. Now what I want to say with this diagram is: if these impulses stop here, that is, if there is no activity of the brain, then, of course, there is no way for the mind to work. If this activity is cut off, as in vigil coma, then after several months the subject is destined for unconsciousness forever, and we can turn off the machine. I agree completely. But I want to know how long and how deep the unconsciousness must be before you turn off the machine. There is no way in which we can turn on the machine again.

A. Lindenmayer (University of Utrecht)

I have a question with regard to the change of probability. How do you visualize this? Is it only local, within the brain? Because if the mind can change the probability in the brain, it can also change the probabilities elsewhere.

J. Eccles

That is a good point, sure! But I am only saying that all this is probabilistic in the microsites here, and there are ten thousand such microsites on one neuron. The mind is not working on one microsite; it is working on the whole ensemble, at a great many microsites on one neuron, and also on adjacent neurons with a similar function. Such amplification is essential. It may be thought, when people see my diagram, that the mind is hovering over here somewhere, where your scalp should be! It is not so at all; it is right within the cortex. That is where the mind is working. We only know its location from where it works. Furthermore the action is reciprocal as is indicated by the reciprocal arrows for mental events in *Figure 12.* I cannot conceive how mental events could be effective elsewhere as in psychokinesis.

W. Kuyk (University of Antwerp)

Can we then separate the mind from the brain? Because there are reasons, for example the Gödel paradox, which suggest that we cannot separate mental events from all the other events. Well, that would be very good for interactionism in a sense, but on the other hand it suggests an ontological unity, and this is how many people take it. There is an emerging movement which looks at the world as being one in the sense that all features are connected. Now I want to know what your reaction is to that.

J. Eccles

I don't like these global, mystical concepts. I just do not want to be immersed in the universal mind all that much! I am an individualist. All my life I have been conscious of my unique existence, and therefore I see everybody else in the same way. I got this consciousness when I was a 17-year-old. I had a vision about myself, and that is why I became a neuroscientist — to understand more and more about how the brain relates to the mind. So I have lived with this feeling of uniqueness. I am a solipsist primarily — if you like, a methodological solipsist. Of course, then we can only know of each other through ourselves. Only because of my own experience do I grant you experiences like I have. And that is the way we should look at humanity, with compassionate love and understanding, for realize that each of you is an embodied being like I am. There is of course a terrible mystery to be discovered — how we come to exist, and so on. I do believe that we are all divine creations. Each of us is an individually created being. That would give us again a global idea, because we are all part of it, we are God's creation. But I think we are still individual existents with our own souls and selves, able to make our decisions up to a point, either for good or evil, just as in the Christian tradition.

B. Gulyás

Sir John, in Descartes' philosophy the brain and the mind (the body and the soul, *res extensa* and *res cogitans*) are on the same ontological level — as "relative substances" — and therefore the interaction between them is a "balanced" interaction, equally effective in both directions.

In your dualist position the brain and the mind are intended to be at the same ontological level, as in the classical Cartesian position. However, in your brain-mind dualism — even if you would like to express your dualist position as a quasi-Cartesian "balanced" dualism — it is not correctly so. Why? Because you frequently point out that there are situations (e.g., vigil coma or other such states) when the mind is still intact while the brain has been damaged. This means the mind still is a self-existing entity on its own, without the brain. And then the mind cannot act any more upon the brain. So they are not on the same ontological level anymore, and there is no room for interaction between them.

J. Eccles

In vigil coma the cerebral cortex may appear normal. It lacks the input from the reticular activating system and so is in deep depression and is unable to react to the mind-coma. But recovery can occur even after many weeks. So brain and mind continued to exist though not interacting. In this dualist interactionism, which Popper and I set up, we give equal status as an entity to the brain or the whole physical world as we do to the mental world. But what we resist is having the mental world, the whole of our conscious ex- periences (World 2), just "pushed" into the brain and made to be a subsidiary component of a reacting brain. That is what we are against. We would like to have two entities: World 1 and World 2. We don't place one above the other: we put them side by side — as interacting. I think it is important to see this interaction, this incredible mystery of existence, as an interaction between self-consciousness and the world. And only through self-consiousness do we know the world at all. So, what comes first is your experience and what follows is your interpretation of it as being a world around you. This is how you learnt as a baby. This is the first thing a baby has to do, even in the mother's uterus, to hear and to act and to appreciate and it goes right on to the beginning of extrauterine life, with vision and so on. We have learnt our world, learnt how to behave, learnt how to appreciate, learnt how to see depths and all the rest of it.

B. Gulyás

I still cannot agree with your explanation, because in your books (e.g., The Self and Its Brain[18], The Human Mystery[7], etc.) you frequently stated that the brain is the result of a long process of biological evolution, while the mind is given to the embryo sometime between conception and birth and is of divine origin. If this is of divine origin and the brain is not, they are not on the same ontological level.

J. Eccles

Let's forget about souls and just take a conscious being, say a cat or a dog or a monkey or a rat, or whatever you like. There is still a World 2, interacting in perception and action with the brain, but they don't have the central core of the self, the knowledge of the world, the future, decision-making knowledge of their value systems, knowledge that they are going to die and all that. That is what we humans have, but I don't think we want to overlook that there is a world of consciousness in animals, and that World 2 for the animal is an entity, with a status equal to World 1 of the brain.

A. Vergote (Catholic University of Leuven)

Sir John, I would like to discuss whether there is not a problem with the definition of interaction. I can understand, as far as I am not a specialist, your argumentation, as I read it in *The Human Psyche*[8]. However the concept of interaction implies, of course, reciprocal causality. And how can you think a causality by the mind on the brain, which would suppose an antecedent existence, a working of the mind, without already involving the working of the brain? For causality, in the strict sense of the world, implies always a temporal sequence.

J. Eccles

But I think we have no evidence. We can assume that there is a temporal sequence, and there has been a lot of work on temporal sequences, by Libet especially on action of the brain and the timing of mental events. We, of course, can only work with one-tenth of a second or that range, but let's keep it open. You want to have a strict identity of time, of simultaneity, strict simultaneity. Now, you think of mental events and brain events as absolutely simultaneous, and therefore they cannot interact. There is no experimental evidence for that. We have to think that we have got time to play in milliseconds, one way or the other. And then the other thing about interaction is, we have it both ways, across the frontier, between brain and mind, the arrows being reciprocal. Always, I think, reciprocity is involved, even on these microsites. And so when you get the mental event changing the frequency of vesicular emission, that goes back also as a signal to the mind. The mind works by causing the signal and registering the effect. Otherwise how would we have experience or perception? How else do we ever know of anything? There has to be a line from the brain to the mind.

O. Creutzfeldt

Aren't we in danger, as often happens in this type of brain-mind discussion, of mixing up categories? Within the probabilistic model, mind has the function of an ill-defined force which has some sort of individuality and which acts as a micro-force on synapses.

Mind as World 3 in the model of Eccles and Popper, on the other hand, is an impersonal world with which an individual can communicate through his brain, like with World 1. It exists and we have access to it by reading books, by referring to ideas, by listening to music or by discussing models of the world. In a narrower sense, this world of the mind is the world of the symbols of the real world and of our experience of it. The brain creates these symbols and understands them. However, the symbols are not isomorphic with the functional structure of the brain, but attempt to be isomorphic with reality.

On the other hand, if we mean by the term "mind" all the capacities of the human brain for reasoning, cognition, planning and action, including the creation of symbols, we define mind differently. It becomes a functional description of the performances of the human brain and here the neurological sciences will lead us far in our understanding.

However, none of these definitions or descriptions *explain* our experience of ourselves or of the world. Why not admit that this is a mystery, and that there is no way of explaining that certain electrochemical activities in certain regions of the brain are "experienced" and others not?

It is a condition of the human mind that it wants to explain everything and develop theories which are complete. These theories are limited by our knowledge of the world.

They developed from magic concepts to our present-day scientific models, but they are always limited by the available knowledge. In his attempt to present complete models, however, man always commits the sin of mixing categories. The world of symbols is related to the real world and our experience of the real world, but neither the symbols nor the experience represent the real world completely. In trying to develop a scientific theory of mind we tend to neglect the fact that mind and matter are different entities, different levels of reality and experience, which may depend on each other, but the analysis of which — as Nicolai Hartmann has pointed out — demands different categories. Any attempts to create complete scientific models of the brain-mind relation, whether based on physical dualism such as John Eccles proposes, or by assuming idealistic superstructures based on monistic theories such as proposed by Sperry or Bunge, are therefore bound to lead into impasses. They have only metaphorical significance.

J. Szentágothai

I would agree with Otto Creutzfeldt up to a certain point. World 3 of Popper is indeed objective if we think of it primarily as written down, say, in a good encyclopedia. It is a world of very complex symbols which we learn to decode. To acquire of a language is to learn to decode a complicated system of strings of phenomena, grammatical, and syntactic rules, etc. — being no linguist I cannot express myself correctly — however, when I understand a certain word and its meaning, it immediately becomes also subjective. Apart from its conventional, everyday meaning, which we use to communicate, each word also has subjective elements attached, some of which are common to people sharing the same cultural background, interest and what not, others are entirely private, linked with one's own private experience. Or are we already entering here World 2 of Popper? It is probably very similar with all other things that we categorize as parts of World 3.

My trouble starts with the consciousness of animals. They

do not have anything like World 3, but they undoubtedly
have some degree of consciousness. Within their specific
ecological spheres, animals — and not only the higher
vertebrates, but also many invertebrates — behave very
intelligently, often as if they had some real insight. Spontaneity, playfulness, and even some aesthetic creativity and
self-purpose — as if "existing" (or behaving) purely for
their own sake — can be seen almost everywhere, down to
very primitive phyla.

Our (more specifically the Christian) belief does not require — in spite of the general assertions to the contrary —
a dualist concept in any Cartesian or neo-Cartesian sense.
This has been made very clear by D.M. MacKay on several
occasions, most concisely in his *Neuroscience* paper "The
Interdependence of Mind and Brain" (on p. 1391)[16]. I have
nothing to add to MacKay's argument. If the Creator is as
revealed in the Bible, there is no incompatibility whatsoever
— against conventional theological and atheistic argumentation — between the belief in resurrection and non-belief
in a dualist philosophy. MacKay's metaphors (or analogies),
taken from modern computer science, have been anticipated
by several thinkers, albeit on a different level (see, for
example, the epitaph Benjamin Franklin composed for himself). I admit that there is a Platonic element in this
reasoning.

J. Eccles

I am not sure what you mean. I absolutely want to defend
the notion of neural machinery. I defend it to the limit as I
also defend my spiritual existence and the reality of the soul
or the self. These are all the realities that I have put in this
diagram — World 1 and World 2 — and the interaction
between them.

J. Szentágothai

And World 3?

J. Eccles

World 3 was a human creation. There was a little World 3 in the Neanderthalian, for example, who had a brain as large as ours, yet had only a most primitive World 3. I am of course a tremendous believer in World 3. But it is not to be confused with the brain-mind problem. From the brain-mind interaction we create World 3 or the understanding of World 3, the appreciation of it, and we can add a little bit of our own to the record of civilization, which is World 3. That is what we do in science. Science is one of the most productive aspects of human creativity today, adding magnificently to World 3. But let us not get confused. My statements claim that there is a World 1, the brain and all its happenings, right down to the ultra-microsites. There is another world, World 2, and don't underestimate the mind. Everybody thinks it is rather fuzzy, but that is because we don't appreciate it enough. As soon as you want to do something, you have to plan it. I want to make a movement; instead of making a messy movement, I can plan a movement to do some specific motor performance, which goes to hundreds of millions of neurons in my sensorimotor area. They must code just the right pattern, and the place to pick up my pencil, and to write then as I wish. It is in my mind in the first place how to plan to do it. It is so for everything we do deliberately, for every skill we have, every expression we make. As I am speaking now to you, I am trying to think how to express myself. All of this is in my mind before I put it into words to talk. And so the mind is rich, beyond any imagining, rich in its structure and in its content and in its memories. I would put memories in the mind in the highest place; the brain carries the data banks. The nearest analogy I can provide is that my mind is like a programmer and my brain is like a computer. I am the programmer, over and above my computer.

W. Kuyk

May I ask you a small question about this point? If it is a human brain that has all these possibilities and, on the other hand, if it is distinguished from the brain of an animal, why don't you put the human brain inside World 3? Because, as I see it, your distinctions of Worlds 1, 2, 3, and so on make the human body less human than the human mind. I would add to this the following question: would it be possible for you, Sir John, to write a book, as you have been doing, on the subject, without using the word "psyche", "mind", "soul", and all such terms, and at the same time say what you want to say?

J. Eccles

The answer is no. I write my books in order to express myself, my own inner declarations; in the words they are wrapped around. All my concepts are wrapped around my central core, my World 2 and my World 3. I am responsible therefore. That is what responsibility means, that you are a self-acting being: criticizing, relating, and all the rest of it. But you are a unique being, central to all of that and responsible for it.

W. Kuyk

May I just extend my question a bit? I am a mathematician by upbringing, and that is why I want to make the following remarks. Yesterday I heard Dr. Creutzfeldt saying that one cannot avoid entirely a dualistic terminology (with emphasis on *terminology*), but he left open the question whether there should be dualist ontology. Now there is a development in mathematics, going on since the thirties, which has changed the whole mathematical world, and is even changing, I believe, a part of the world of physics. It started with Kurt Gödel. Of course, we have this famous book by Douglas Hofstadter, *Gödel, Escher, Bach*[12], and I

think what the author wants to do in the book is to explain
to all of us, to all the public, what really happened in
mathematics. I do think that the main point of the book is
still quite difficult for many people, non-mathematicians, to
understand. The main point, as mathematicians see it nowadays, is that Gödel discovered that as soon as a language
system or a sentence that is supposed to carry semantical
meaning, as soon as that sentence or that system becomes
self-referential, then it is bound to give rise to contradictions, to paradoxes. And I think if you speak about the brain
or if you say I think about thinking, then you are definitly
being self-referential. And of course the implication is, if
you think about your own thinking, you are more apt to get
into contradictions than when you think about the thinking
of other people.

   Now my point is: is it not so that all the discussions that
are going on about the brain-mind problem and the kind of
contradictions that they engender, especially when people of
the same basic mind, the same basic mentality, talk about
it, are similar to those that took place in mathematics, let us
say before 1930? Nowadays mathematicians aren't as easily
trapped by paradoxes since they have ways of avoiding self-
referentiality. And so what happens in mathematics and
logic is that we create all kinds of local systems that exclude
every self-referentiality, (the word "local" meaning that all
these systems have only a limited range of applicability and
meaning). That is to say, if we follow this line, it could well
be that in science, in humanities, in philosphy, we do not
get further than making local systems that have validity
only up to a certain point, and we may try to link these
little theories up to each other. But in doing so we may lose
connections in other regions, so that we have, so to speak, a
broken kind of science, which consists of all kinds of not
entirely compatible subsystems.

   All this does not mean that one may not speak about the
"self", the "soul", the "mind", etc., by way of poetic
language, love language, faith language, theological language, body language, etc., thus in terms that have no
sharply defined (but rather a "holistic") meaning, and
where paradoxes are "legal". Inasmuch as even these holis-

tic languages should not be put on a par and mixed, one
should certainly not use any of them mixed with scientific
language, which is unequivocal and by definition consistent.
In the philosophy of man, the choice seems to be between,
on the one hand, using a language which holds on to the
unity of man (at the expense of having to deal with him in
terms of a great number of not entirely compatible but
complementary scientific languages), and, on the other
hand, mixing scientific and holistic language into one
blend, with the hope that this blend may become consistent
one day (but at the expense of having to split man into body
and soul, consigning the two to the separate Worlds, 1 and
2 respectively). The quantum dynamic approach, as mentioned in Sir John Eccles' lecture and suggested by Margenau
seems to support the first choice rather than the latter. For
instance, the essence of the wave versus particle complementarity is the *unity of the two and not their interaction* (interaction
takes place between wave packets, i.e., between particles, as
such). Complementarity is the expression of the impossi-
bility of bringing together into one perceptual framework (and into one (scientific) language system) what
happens at the microphysical level, forcing us to conceive of
wave packets as probability functions. Thus, if particles
correspond to perceptible (but not necessarily conscious)
events (such as somatosensory sensation, a thought, or the
contraction of a particular muscle), riding on the waves of
the nervous system, and, moreover, if wave packets are
probability packets of the same, then one should look for
"Heisenberg pairs" of properties of events that are related
by uncertainty. I suggest that the following is an example:
the "higher" the type of event, the more imprecise is its
cerebral substrate defined, i.e., the more globally is that
substrate distributed. Here, the word "higher" is to be
taken in the sense of ascending from the vital type of
functions (body motion, rhythms, instincts, etc.) up to the
emotional, psychic, rational, aesthetic, moral, and religious
ones. The word "substrate" denotes the underlying cerebral
system of neuronal subnetworks that is being "fired" when
the event is "on". From this perspective, the various forms
of sleeping and unconsciousness correspond to various forms

of a vacuum: there is always wave activity going on with the possibility of protons (and antiprotons) appearing and disappearing (compare with the REM sleep and its accompanying dreams), just as a "quantum theory of the brain" deals a blow to reductionism and various forms of materialism.

O. Creutzfeldt

The Gödel argument as you applied it to our discussion would indicate that reason as a system of symbols with semantic meanings will lead to contradictions and paradoxes when trying to analyse the nature of reason. I agree with that and this is, in fact, contained in the words of Kant which I quoted in my lecture about the nature of reason, which asks questions about itself which it cannot answer. This argument does not relate necessarily to the brain-mind problem as such, however. Here we ask whether the working of the brain is sufficient to explain our models of thinking, reasoning, beliefs and concepts.

I think we are all convinced that the brain is the necessary condition for mind and reason as far as it is accessible to man. I wanted to point out, however, that brain mechanisms cannot offer a sufficient explanation of mind and reason. The ability of our brains to create symbols of reality, its symbolic competence, is the basic condition. However, the whole system of symbols, their logical connections, are no longer a function of our brain. Rather, our linguistic symbols and the grammar which connects them, must be as consistent as possible with the reality of the world around us and with our experience, which they try to represent. I consider it as a mistake in linguistics to conclude that the postulated general grammar reflects the functional structure of the brain. Instead, the general grammar is dictated by the reality of the world and the objects in it which the language tries to describe in symbolic signals, i.e., words. These words have to be related to each other in a way that is consistent with the way in which the objects it describes are related to each other in our experience.

J. Szentágothai

Let us return to the question whether self-referential reasoning, unavoidable wherever mind tries to explore mind, would not get us into difficulties foreseen by Gödel's theorem. Gödel's theorems state — as I am able to understand from the secondary literature — that every system of axioms has certain propositions that can neither be proven nor falsified within the framework of that very system of axioms. Although the limits of formal mathematics were defined by formal mathematical arguments, these limits cannot be so rigidly observed in "non-formal" mathematics. As demonstrated by Lakatos[14], non-formal mathematics is qualified in the sense of Karl Popper as a scientific discipline which emerges from the competition and cooperation of theories and *not* by deductive arguments of formalized mathematics.

Both natural brains and artificial computing devices are capable of executing symbol manipulations, and hence may qualify as being self-referential. The conceptual and methodological gap between "non-formal" theories of brains and computers is still very wide, but it is likely that emergent knowledge in neurobiology will be able to give important new clues for the design of new types of computing devices. In view of the newly recognized recursivity and repeated reentrance in nervous systems — supported by the mentioned fact that about 80-90% of all connections of the cerebral cortex are cortico-cortical — the neural systems can be considered as quasi-closed neuronal networks, in which internal structure, shape, and relative positions of neurons determine the domain of possible brain states.

A rather extreme approach to neurobiological computations is based on a connectionist model[1]. At least a part of the brain can be modeled as a "connectionist computer" suited for parallel problem solving. The power of biological computation is limited by a trade-off principle[5]: a system cannot at the same time be effectively programmable, amenable to evolution by variation and selection, and computationally efficient. Further research on the possibility of building newer generations of computing devices utilizing our knowledge and ideas about the organizational principles of the nervous system could better illuminate the computational capabilities of the brain as well as their limits, in the spirit of Gödel's theorems, and of the Church-Turing thesis emphasizing the role of algorithms instead of axioms.

H. Roelants (Catholic University of Leuven)

I want to come back to the first intervention of Professor Creutzfeldt and ask a question in that connection: I think that under the name "brain-mind problem" very different questions can be referred to, e.g., one important question is certainly that of individuality (or personal identity). But perhaps other questions are equally important concerning the brain-mind problem and, in my opinion, the most central question concerns *the causal efficacy of symbols,* and that which is sometimes called the *symbolic order.* I would like to know the position of the three invited speakers on that. How far do they agree that the problem of how symbols can have causal efficacy is the central problem of what we call the brain-mind problem? And when I use the term "causal efficacy of symbols" I take it in a very general sense, including the all-pervasive domain of suggestions, of the influence of verbal and other symbols in some kinds of therapies, and in life in general.

This has something to do with the causal efficacy of what Karl Popper calls World 3, but perhaps it is not completely the same. Personally, I do not think that we have at this moment a satisfactory theory even of what a symbol is, and I certainly do not think we have a satisfactory theory of how symbols can have causal efficacy.

O. Creutzfeldt

Symbols have, of course, a causal efficacy. If we talk with each other, we use linguistic signals as symbols. These symbols relate to and describe a reality, but are not this reality itself. Nevertheless, they affect our perception of the world, our thinking and action. On a more complex level, any theory about the world which we accept, be it a mythological or a scientific model, has an effect on us. In this sense, symbols are a reality, a conceptual reality, one may say. This applies also to physical theories of matter, such as the theory of atoms, which only describes what we can measure (or falsify). These theories influence our mind by leading to further measurements, and have to be adjusted or completely changed if the new measurements reveal new facts which cannot be fit into the old model.

The cognitive sciences and epistemology are concerned with the relation between our ideas, or symbols, and the reality which they are supposed to represent. Without the ability and capacity for symbols, without the symbolic competence of the human brain, there would be no mind to think about. Therefore, I cannot imagine an animal having a mind in the sense we are speaking of.

J. Eccles

I would agree with that. Just take an experience for a moment: while you were talking, I was thinking about what you were saying and what the meaning was. Now I put it into language; I have to try to say this thing. As soon as it is put into language, it is a symbol. But I don't know how widely you want to use the word "symbol". You didn't define it. So I think it is an open-ended kind of operation. Let's think of what we are doing all the time: we have thoughts, we are expressing and criticizing them, we are writing them out. We read and criticize and imagine into the future. I think that one of the great skills is imagination; you may imagine in symbols. I don't know whether you imagine so much in symbols. You imagine in situations, dynamic situations. A lot of our imagination is in a dynamic manner and into the future, into planning, into what you will do tomorrow and so on. All of this, and then going over to do your planning, and so on. We are living in a very complex world which is not only the present and the past but also the future. And that is where ordinary animals fail completely. They have no imagination of the future. That is something that has come with the development of the brain and self-consciousness. I do believe in the humanoid story. In some way, which I think is a divine intervention, when humanoids got to certain levels of performance — and Popper thinks it is a miracle also — they became self-conscious beings, each carrying a self at the core of its being. That is what has been given the whole of civilization, because those selves started to create, working selectively and with imagination in the world: stone axes and paintings on the walls of their caves, and so on. With language which would already have been developed (we don't know when and how) eventually the high civilizations came, first in Sumer. And this is straight on to us — this is World 3. But this came through creating selves. We have to think about the mystery of being. So I think that each of us is a miracle. And we have to think about the divine creation. We are part of it. That is my only explanation of how I came to be, how you came to be, having as our home planet Earth, all our world with all of its wonderful beauty.

H. Roelants

There is a second part to my question. I think that the questions, "what is a symbol?" and "how can it have causal efficacy?" can eventually be formulated, at least partly, as scientific problems. We will perhaps have to wait a very long time before we have a satisfactory theory giving answers, but do you think such a scientific theory is in principle possible?

J. Eccles

I don't think that empirical science should be extended in that direction. You cannot investigate that scientifically. That is in the sphere of the philosophy of science. Let us keep science for a fairly strict compartment of human activity, so that we do not intrude beyond our sphere. I want to resist the reductionist, who wants to reduce everything down, further and further.

H. Roelants

But an explanation need not necessarily be a reduction.

J. Eccles

It is a reduction to say that all problems are in principle scientific.

H. Roelants

That is another thing.

J. Eccles

You just cannot handle the older value systems in a scientific way. You have your own philosophy, you have your own beliefs. You don't know how to put up an empirical experiment falsifying it in the Popperian manner. You have to test by explanatory power, absence of self-contradiction and all those kinds of criteria.

J. Szentágothai

The question raised by Professor Roelants is most exciting, and I would have very little to add to, or disagree with, what has been said by either Otto Creutzfeldt or by Sir John Eccles. What I am particularly amazed by is that we can simultaneously manipulate and process very different systems of symbols; while talking or listening to others' talking I can also look around in this audience and can take note of some details in my visual field, an interesting face or colour composition of clothing — especially in the ladies, i.e., something irrelevant for the problem in the center of our attention — and yet this does not interfere too much with the main mental work. Julius Caesar and also Napoleon were reputedly able to dictate letters simultaneously to 5 or 6 different scribes on a variety of very important subjects. Splitting our attention in a cross-talk around the table is a very common ability, and yet it requires one to use the same word (symbol) with very different meanings according to the specific context. In the case of a master chess player who plays blind simultaneously against a number of opponents, it is usually claimed that when each opponent pronounces his next move the master can recreate backwards the mental image of the position and his specific strategy that he had used and has to further develop. Here advantage is taken, obviously, of some kind of time-sharing ability, stowing away for various segments of time one piece in order to deal with the other.

The same problem comes up in the observation of "split-brain" patients. Originally, it was assumed that the right hemisphere, in the vast majority of people, is practically mute. However, when Zaidel[23] used an occluder attached to the eyes by contact lenses, and objects or patterns could be scanned for longer periods by either hemisphere, it turned out that the right hemisphere also has a vocabulary, although organized in a different mode: a convention-bound template-matching, rather than the syntactic and phonetic analysis by the left hemisphere. The question is now how we use the two kinds of vocabulary and processing, as in fast reading and in the processing of spoken language.

This touches upon the fundamental question of the unity of consciousness. Although each of us can divide our attention among several, simultaneously occurring things, both perceived and in the process of being executed, we do not feel any split in our consciousness as a single self. Donald and Valerie MacKay (reported more extensively by D.M. MacKay[17]) have tried in several of Sperry's "split brain" cases to find any clear proof of disproof of two separate consciousnesses. Eventually they had to give up because neither was convincing. It is also well known and vividly described by many authors that in extreme situations — during accidents, catastrophes, great personal danger, upon being notified of something dreadful that has happened or is about to happen to oneself or someone close to us — the person involved has the experience of being at once the subject and an external observer of the events. But I do not think that all this is of much use for unraveling the relation between brain and mind.

H. De Dijn (Catholic University of Leuven)

I would like to ask a question of Professor Creutzfeldt. For some reason, man spontaneously and inevitably thinks about himself using a dualistic terminology. In this thinking of himself he inevitably uses symbols like "soul", "person", "daughter of somebody", "husband", "wife", "somebody having a destiny, responsibility", and so on. On the other hand, we also talk about ourselves in a purely objectifying way, which takes on a special, elaborated form in science. Now I would like to ask you whether you would agree that this has certain consequences for the relationship between philosophy and science.

Philosophy; what can it say about the significance of the scientific picture for the way man consciously lives himself in a symbolic way? Philosophy could be the analysis of the organization of the symbols in which man spontaneously and inevitably lives. Philosophical discussion, as I understand it, starts from this way we symbolically live ourselves, and I think this discussion itself has shown that the interest in the theme itself starts from there and can only be understood from there. It is, in other words, inevitably related to — it cannot be purely scientific probably — moral and ideological questions, which precisely belong to this symbolic way people live themselves. That is my question: aren't discussions like these philosophical through and through, and not scientific?

I have a remark as well, again related to what you said in this discussion. You said that your position is not necessarily a reductionism. The symbolic way we inevitably see ourselves, as you said, is still a reality; I think you said "a conceptual reality". I understand that to mean that it is not a reality to be discovered and tested empirically. But then of course the question arises: how can we still call this a reality? My suggestion would be (and again, I would like to ask your opinion about this) that it is a reality in the sense that we care about it, and everything we care about is, of course, in a certain sense, a reality. And it is very clear that we can and do care about many things which are purely symbolic. For example, we even care about fiction.

O. Creutzfeldt

This is a philosophical question. However, we should not fall into the semantic trap which the English use of the word 'science' (i.e., 'physics') as opposed to 'humanities' (i.e., 'philosophy') might suggest. This dichotomy brings with it a challenge for some philosophers such as Feigl, Ryle or Bunge; they feel it necessary to reduce mind and reason to brain mechanisms. However, causality is not restricted to physics, although different causal laws may apply to the different levels of reality as Nicolai Hartmann and Richard Jung have pointed out. The reduction of mind and reason to the physical laws on which they rest and to which they relate is not necessary as a proof of their reality, and can, in fact, never render a sufficient proof as I tried to point out in my lecture.

With reference to our discussion, it is clear that symbols are a reality inasmuch they affect our life and we care about them. Scientific (physical) theories make us understand the causal connections between things. They are necessarily reductionistic. The human mind is not satisfied by them, however. Man wants explanations of the purposes of things. Therefore, even in scientific theories, teleological arguments cannot be avoided. The evolutionary theory, for example, is essentially a teleological concept. There are wider and wider concepts which attempt to explain the purpose of our lives, of history, etc. The broadest of such concepts is "God", in whom — for a religious person — everything rests, and who provides for all the explanations man is looking for. Scientific models, which are also only symbols of reality, are important and determine our lives, no matter whether we know it or not, and no matter whether we accept it or not. They give us a limited view of the world, but they neither answer all the questions we are asking nor explain the purpose of things or of our lives. No ethical principles and therefore no moral arguments or moral postulates can be deduced from scientific explanations as such. For that, higher purposes and goals are needed: humanitarian, social, religious or political goals, which are based on concepts of man and society, of the relation between the individual and God, or on utopian social ideals, respectively. None of these can be proven or determined scientifically (or in physical terms), however.

L. Bencze (Eötvös University, Budapest)

I think St. Thomas Aquinas was fully aware of the problems which we are talking about here, when he, as a philosopher, made a clear distinction between "soul" and "body", or in today's vocabulary "mind" and "brain". Then he went on as a scientist and said mind/soul doesn't exist without brain/body. Then, as a theologian and believer, he went on again and said yes, but as a believer I must say that God provides a certain force for the soul to exist later, for a short time without a body, or separated from the body but such existence is not in accord with its nature (*Summa Theologiae,* I, q. 89, a. 1, resp.). Then, at the resurrection, soul and body will be united, but not the way they existed in this life. So, I think he was very cautious — and a genius at the same time — not to be condemned by the Church for being a heretic, according to its terms. Yet, he emphasized that soul/mind does not exist without brain/body. And I think in this way he was a scientist as well.

O. Creutzfeldt

This is, of course, his Aristotelian tradition. For Aristotle *anima, pneuma,* the soul is related to the body like form to matter. This is a very nice metaphor. Form does not exist without matter in which it can express itself. And matter, the body, on the other hand, cannot become what it is, a mindful matter, without this form. It is of significance, in this context, that the Christian dogma implies the resurrection of the body, because the person is nonexistent without mind *and* body. Other religions assume rebirth in another body, reincarnation, etc. These are all wonderful metaphors that give one a fascinating insight into the mystical relationship between mind and body as man sees it. However, if one wishes to avoid mysticism, it is better to remain on the ground of science and to admit that there is more to be explained about our world than scientific models can offer.

M. Nauwelaerts (Leuven)

Professor Creutzfeldt, do I understand your viewpoint correctly if I formulate it in the words of Immanuel Kant, who spoke about the *"Grenzen der Erkenntnis"*. You say: well, you have science and then you can come to a certain point, and beyond that point you come into the region of believing, into the region of theology, or something like that, and you don't see it as possible that there is any link — a scientific link — between them.

O. Creutzfeldt

Yes, I am afraid that this is so. If one starts to mix up these two worlds of thinking, one soon gets into impasses and paradoxes, if not into obscure occultism. Thus, if one assumes that "mind" is a physical force such as magnetism or gravitation, one soon will end up in strange, chimerical theories. This is the reason, Sir John, why I personally object to your kind of dualistic theory. Once you accept mind as a physical force, you must ask the next question — and you are courageous enough to do it — where it interacts with the brain, where the liaison is, and finally you have to answer the question what the (physical) nature of mind is. Also, if one identifies God with a physical force, one must develop a physical system in which this god-force can be identified and measured. It was the great accomplishment of Thomas Aquinas to try to unite the physical and the metaphysical, but his beautiful scholastic world stands on earthen feet as long as the physical nature of God cannot be proven. If God is identified with a physical force, he is but a force and thus not God anymore. This argument can also be applied, *ceteris paribus,* to the brain-mind discussion, which is therefore a metaphysical question.

Yet as man wants to understand the world and needs to locate himself within a larger context, he will always ask questions about the significance, the meaning, the sense of life *(Sinn des Lebens).* And he will always find the answer in an *ultimum movens,* be it God or a substitute, an idol. One should realize, however, that this leads us into another realm, into another way of looking at the world than looking through the eyes of a scientist.

J. Eccles

I would like to come in and say a few thing at this stage. I am always wanting to make precise statements, to get precise thinking which can be tested in one way and developed from all that. And the story I was putting forth yesterday I think has not been appreciated in the sense that I use a microsite theory for the operation of mental events and neural events. If you once can get that one operation, neuroscience will give you the rest, as global as you want. That is the point that I made yesterday. Now another point: when it comes to the very nature of the self, we have a long lifetime. Each of us is aware, of course, that we are created with genes, with a lot of epigenetic operations as well. The genes work with the many secondary instructions, the Waddington environmental landscape, and so go on to build a human being. That is the baby's brain, where the whole of nature comes in. The nurture is what you do the whole of life: learning, learning and learning. So there are in us components both of nature and nurture. A lot of people are devoted to nature: everything is in the genes; others are devoted to nurture: everything is in the learning. They are both wrong. We are dual and our whole life story has been in that way.

The final point I want to make is this: let's think about the cosmos and the beginning of it all. I wrote a book, *The Human Mystery*[7], on that subject, from the big bang onwards. And there is a story which is relevant to this. We have the anthropic principle. This is what cosmological scientists are talking about. There is also a book just out by Barrow and Tipler[2]. And there is consideration of the physical constants and the size of the original big cosmological bang. Everything seems to have been designed, in the minutest detail, in order to give rise to a cosmos in which our solar system could come to be, with the right kind of minerals, with the right environment and atmosphere for life to begin. So, life could begin to evolve and then we go to the whole of evolution, and here we are. This is the anthropic principle: the cosmos was made so that we could come to exist. Isn't that an extraordinary statement for scientists to make? A teleological statement, to a degree! Let's forget about Monod. We have to believe in teleology, we have to believe that there is design — and I think divine design — in the whole cosmos. And this is what essentially the *anthropic principle* is. That is the most challenging concept.

M. Astroh (Wolfson College, Oxford)

I would like to recall the example of a couple in California that deprived its child of any cultural education. It was nearly impossible to integrate this human being into a social form of human life, for there seemed to be no criteria with which to decide whether it had acquired a self. Leaving aside the difficult ethical problem as to what extent this unfortunate child is to be treated as a human creature, I would like to know more about the evolutionary aspects of the acquisition of the self in both an onto- and a phylogenetic sense.

J. Szentágothai

I am afraid that we know next to nothing about how the self is acquired. Since we are inclined to equate human self-awareness with speech — at least in the first approximation — the best approach would be to analyze the development of language. Complete or virtually complete deprivation of human contact can result from two different causes: children reared by animals, or deprived by criminal neglect and/or mistreatment by their environment. The case I have mentioned belongs to the second category: the case of "Genie" (a pseudonym in order to shield the identity of the victim who still has some further potential to develop) is, so far, the only case that is undoubtedly genuine and scientifically well-documented[6]. The first category was — and still is — considered legendary. These are the so called "wolf children" about whom many stories have become known from antiquity, the Middle Ages, and even from 17th-18th century Europe. Although it is hard to believe, the case of the two Midnapore (India) children is unquestionably true[19] concerning the main facts, reasonably well-documented by the Rev. J.A.L. Singh both by a diary and about forty-odd poor, but still sufficiently clear, photographic snapshots. What has been criticized with certain justification in the story of Rev. Singh are some naive Lamarckian assumptions about changes of the limbs and jaws thought to be caused by the quadrupedal gait of the children and their feeding on the usual prey of wolves. These assumptions are clearly not supported by the photographs. As it appears from the thorough study of R.M. Zingg, such cases may not be rare in India, due to the practice by primitive aboriginal tribes of abandoning especially female children in early infancy, and to some ecological opportunity arising from the behaviour of a subspecies of wolves endemic in India.

The considerable material gathered by R.M. Zingg on both European and Indian wild children is at little variance with the recent and scientifically studied case of "Genie". Such "wolf" or "wild children" appear to be completely "inhuman" when first found, and it takes years of patience and loving care to achieve even a very modest rehabilitation. They can rarely if ever go beyond 20-80 simple words that are never used spontaneously, but only in response to questions and elicited upon command and often require some coercion. From the psycholinguistically-studied case of Genie it appears that speech is processed by the right hemisphere, which would correspond to the assumption[15] that the built-in neural apparatus of the left hemisphere for speech acquisition has long passed its critical period.

There is some evidence that children raised in virtual isolation by a deaf-mute grandparent may develop and communicate in some private language. Such cases as reported by Jespersen[13] are usually not unequivocal, because by the time they could be studied by a competent observer, such children have learned to dissimulate and are quickly acquiring normal speech from their environment. In spite of this, some extremely interesting syntactic rules were observed that do not exist in any contemporary European language but did exist in ancient European languages, like double and triple use of the same word of negation (i.e., not like "*ne ... pas*" in French). It is probably safe to assume that any isolated group of humans would very quickly develop some language with a sophisticated vocabulary, grammatical and syntactic rules[10,11]. The well-known fact that where geographical circumstances prevent communication between closely neighbouring populations (tropical rain forests, high mountain ranges) entirely different languages are developed, also points in this direction. The ability for communication by spoken language is built-in anatomically in the human brain, probably largely in the so-called *planum temporale* on the upper surface of the temporal lobe, where significant differences of cortical surface, left over right, have been observed by Geschwind and Levitsky[9]. In our own unpublished double-blind study of 10 human adult brains a sterological analysis (for cortical volume, cell numbers and cell density) has revealed a 30% difference of left > right.

Unfortunately this does not tell us anything about how human language and hence experience of self-awareness might have arisen. We have to accept its existence as a mystery, but a mystery that seems to have a highly-developed anatomical apparatus (and obviously corresponding physiological functions) as its basis.

A. László (Brussels)

Sir John, I think that in the realm of this discussion of the brain-mind problem one of the main questions is the vantage point that we usually use to approach things. We conceive ourselves as persons with mind, brain, soul, heart. We also conceive ourselves as personalities. These, in my point of view, are restricted-focus images, pictures we carry with ourselves and which we always use to interpret other things in the world. Perhaps I can use an image to throw light upon another possible point of view. When one sees a wave emerging out of the ocean, one can look upon this wave as a wave that is emerging. One can also have another vantage point, that the whole ocean is emerging in that wave. So holistically speaking — you said that the cosmos was made so that we can exist — I would like to add, if you allow: isn't it a miracle that we can participate in this process of creation, that all beings can participate in this miracle?

J. Eccles

Of course, I agree completely with you. I should say that this cosmological principle is not the anthropic principle of Barrow and Tipler. I read very quickly through their book and they keep out all religious meanings from their teleology. They try to be hard scientists and that really means to me that it is meaningless in the end. We have to think that if we are coming to exist, there must be purpose and meaning in this cosmos that gives us our existence. That is,

I would say, teleology. So I agree with you: ultimately everything is miraculous. Each of us is a miraculous creation. And we have to think of the whole cosmos as being likewise. That is, of course, my answer to the reductionists. They cannot even explain themselves and their coming to be.

M. Callens (Catholic University of Leuven)

You will agree with me that we have had a very interesting conference on the brain-mind problem, and it is certainly due to three eminent speakers: Sir John Eccles, Dr. Szentágothai and Dr. Creutzfeldt, whom I thank on your behalf. We are perhaps a little bit sad — and glad, at the same time — because we didn't solve the complete problem, but we are left with something to think about.

REFERENCES

1. BALLARD, D.H. (1986). Cortical Connections and Parallel Processing: Structure and Function. *Behav. Brain. Sci.* 9: 67-120.
2. BARROW, J.D. and TIPLER, F.J. (1986). *The Anthropic Cosmological Principle.* Oxford: Clarendon Press.
3. BUNGE, M. (1977). Emergence and the Mind. *Neuroscience* 2: 501-509.
4. CHANGEUX, J.-P. (1983). *L'homme neuronal.* Paris: Fayard. See also HEIDMANN, A., HEIDMANN, Th. and J.-P. CHANGEUX (1984), *C.R. Acad. Sci.* Paris 299, Serie III. 839-844.
5. CONRAD, M. (1985). On Design Principles of Molecular Computers. *Comm. ACM* 28: 464-480.
6. CURTISS, Susan (1977). *Genie: A Psycholinguistic Study of a Modern Day "Wild Child".* New York: Academic Press.
7. ECCLES, J.C. (1979). *The Human Mystery.* (Gifford Lectures for 1978). Berlin-Heidelberg-New York: Springer.
8. ECCLES, J.C. (1980). *The Human Psyche.* (Gifford Lectures for 1979). Berlin-Heidelberg-New York: Springer.
9. GESCHWIND, N. and LEVITSKY, W. (1968). Human Brain: Left-right Assymetrics in Temporal Speach Region. *Science* 161: 186-187.
10. HALE, A. (1886). The Origin of Languages. *Amer. Ass. for Advancement of Sci.* 35.
11. HALE, A. (1888). *The Development of Language.* Toronto: Canadian Institute.
12. HOFSTADTER, D.R. (1979). *Gödel, Escher, Bach: An Eternal Golden Braid.* New York: The Harvester Press.
13. JESPERSSEN, O. (1922 [1925]). *Language, its Nature, Development, and Origin,* London. German translation. *Die Sprache, ihre Natur, Entwicklung und Entstehung.* Heidelberg: Carl Winters Univ. Buchhandlung, 1925.
14. LAKATOS, J. (1970). Falsification and the Methodology of Scientific Research Programmes. In: *Criticism and the Growth of Knowledge,* J. LAKATOS and MUSGRAVE, (eds.). London: Cambridge University Press.
15. LENNEBERG, E.H. (1967). *Biological Foundations of Language.* New York: John Wiley and Sons.
16. MacKAY, D.M. (1980). The Interdependence of Mind and Brain. *Neuroscience* 5: 1389-1391.
17. MacKAY, D.M. (1981). Neural Basis of Cognitive Experience. *Adv. Physiol. Sci.* vol. 30. In: Neural Communication and Control, SZÉKELY, Gy.; LÁBOS, E., DAMJANOVICH, S. (eds.). Oxford-Budapest: Pergamon Press-Akadémiai Kiadó, pp. 315-332.
18. POPPER, K.R. and ECCLES, J.C. (1977). *The Self and Its Brain.* Berlin-Heidelberg-New-York: Springer.

19. SINGH, the Rev. J.A.L. and ZINGG, R.M. (1939 [1941, 1942 repr.]). *Wolf-Children and Feral Man*. New York and London: Harper and Brothers Publishers.
20. SPERRY, W.R. (1980). Mind-Brain Interaction: Mentalism, Yes; Dualism, No. *Neuroscience* 5: 195-206.
21. SZENTÁGOTHAI, J. (1984). Downward Causation?. *Ann. Rev. Neurosci.* 7: 1-11.
22. WITELSON, S.F. and PALLIE, W. (1973). Left Hemisphere Specialization for Language in the Newborn. *Brain* 96: 641-646.
23. ZAIDEL, E. (1978). Lexical Organization in the Right Hemisphere. In: *Cerebral Correlates of Conscious Experience*, BUSER, P.A. and ROUGEUL-BUSER, A. (eds.), Amsterdam: Elsevier-North Holland. INSERM SYMPOS 6: 177-197, and Concepts of Cerebral Dominance in the Split Brain, *ibid.* 263-284.

SOME PREVIOUS PUBLICATIONS
CONCERNING THE BRAIN-MIND PROBLEM
BY THE SAME AUTHORS

O. CREUTZFELDT

1975. Neurophysiological Correlates of Different Functional States of the Brain. In: *Brain Work*, Alfred Benzon Symposium, Munksgaard, pp. 21-47.

1977. Physiological Conditions of Consciousness. In: *Wld. Congr. Neurol.*, DEN HARTOG JAGER, W.A., *et al.*, (eds.). I.C.S., no. 434, Excerpta Medica, Amsterdam, pp. 194-208.

1979. Neurophysiological Mechanisms and Consciousness. In: *Brain and Mind.* CIBA Foundation Symposion 69 (New Series). Excerpta Medica, Amsterdam, pp. 217-233.

1981a. Philosophische Probleme der Neurophysiologie. In: *Rückblick in die Zukunft*, H. ROESNER (ed.). Berlin: Severin und Siedler, pp. 256-278.

1981b. Diversification and Synthesis of Sensory Systems across the Cortical Link. In: *Brain Mechanisms of Perceptual Awareness and Purposeful Behavior*, O. POMPEIANO and C. AJMONE-MARSAN (eds.). New York: Raven Press, pp. 153-166.

1983. *Cortex Cerebri.* Berlin-Heidelberg-New York: Springer.

1984. Impasses and Fallacies of the Brain-Mind Discussion. *Exp. Brain Res. Suppl.* 9: 33-41.

1986. Gehirn und Geist. In: *Bursfelder Universitätsreden.* L. PERLITT (ed.). Göttingen: Göttinger Tageblatt Verlag.

J.C. ECCLES

1953. *The Neurophysiological Basis of Mind: The Principles of Neurophysiology*, (Waynflete Lectures 1952). Oxford: Clarendon Press.

1966. *Brain and Conscious Experience*, (Conference of the Pontifical Academy of Sciences 1964). Berlin-Heidelberg-New York: Springer.

1970. *Facing Reality*. Berlin-Heidelberg-New York: Springer.

1973. *The Understanding of the Brain*, (Patten Lectures 1972). New York: Mc-Graw Hill.

1977. *The Self and Its Brain* (with K. POPPER). Berlin-Heidelberg-New York: Springer.

1979. *The Human Mystery*, (Gifford Lectures 1978). Berlin-Heidelberg-New York: Springer.

1980. *The Human Psyche*, (Gifford Lectures 1979). Berlin-Heidelberg-New York: Springer.

1980. *Gehirn und Geist* (with H. ZEIER). München: Kindler.

1984. *The Wonder of Being Human: Our Brain, Our Mind* (with D.N. ROBINSON). New York: Free Press.